TOPICS IN Language Disorders

Language Disorders of Hearing-Impaired Children

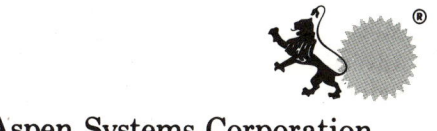

Aspen Systems Corporation

TLD
Topics In Language Disorders

An Aspen Publication®

Publisher: John R. Marozsan
Editorial Director: R. Curtis Whitesel
Managing Editor: Margot S. Raphael
Associate Editor: Barbara R. Richman

Editorial Assistant: Emily L. Scott
Production Manager: Paul R. Carlin
Manager Fulfillment Operations:
  Ernest V. Manzella, Jr.

TOPICS IN LANGUAGE DISORDERS (USPS 597-090) is published quarterly by Aspen Systems Corporation, 16792 Oakmont Avenue, Gaithersburg, MD 20877. Second-class postage paid at Gaithersburg, Maryland and additional mailing offices. POSTMASTER: Send address changes to Aspen Systems Corporation, 16792 Oakmont Avenue, Gaithersburg, MD 20877.

Subscription rates: $42.00 per year in the United States and Canada (four issues). Payable in advance. Subscribers may specify a particular issue to begin the subscription if desired. **Subscribers in the United Kingdom, Europe, Middle East, and Africa:** Address subscription inquiries to Costello, 43 The High Street, Tunbridge Wells, Kent TN1 1XU, England. **Subscribers in Japan** address subscription inquiries to Maruzen Company, Ltd., P.O. Box 5050, Tokyo International, 100-31, JAPAN.

Editorial correspondence (letters to the editor and manuscript submissions) should be addressed to: Editorial Director, TLD, Aspen Systems Corporation, 1600 Research Boulevard, Rockville, MD 20850.

Business correspondence (subscription inquiries, subscription orders, change of address, etc.) should be addressed to Fulfillment Operations, Aspen Systems Corporation, 16792 Oakmont Avenue, Gaithersburg, MD 20877.

Notices for change of address, including the subscriber's old and new addresses, should be sent to Fulfillment Operations, Aspen Systems Corporation, 16792 Oakmont Avenue, Gaithersburg, MD 20877 6 weeks in advance of effective date.

Single Copies: $13.00 each; enclose payment with order. **Multiple Copies for Educational and Training Programs:** Inquiries from bona fide educational programs concerning terms of sale will be answered promptly. Send inquiries to: Fulfillment Operations, Aspen Systems Corporation, 16792 Oakmont Avenue, Gaithersburg, MD 20877.

Advertising: Direct inquiries and correspondence to Journal Advertising Sales, Department 4A, Aspen Systems Corporation, 1600 Research Boulevard, Rockville, MD 20850. Telephone: (301) 251-5000.

Copyright © 1982 by Aspen Systems Corporation, 1600 Research Boulevard, Rockville, Maryland 20850. All rights reserved.

Microform: This publication is available in microform from University Microfilms International, 300 North Zeeb Road, Dept. P.R., Ann Arbor, MI 48106. Article reprints are also available from University Microfilms International, Article Reprint Service, at the same address.

Permission to copy: The appearance of the code at the bottom of the first page of an article in this journal indicates the copyright owner's consent that copies of the article may be made for personal or internal use, or for the personal or internal use of specific clients. **This consent is given on the condition, however, that the copier pay the stated per-copy fee through the Copyright Clearance Center, Inc. for copying beyond that permitted by Section 107 or 108 of the U.S. Copyright Law.** Send article code, the number of copies made, and payment (for cost per copy, see the last four digits of the code) to: Copyright Clearance Center, Inc., 21 Congress St., Salem, MA 01970.

This consent does not extend to other kinds of copying, such as copying for general distribution, for advertising or promotional purposes, for creating new collective works, or for resale.

"This publication is designed to provide accurate and authoritative information in regard to the Subject Matter covered. It is sold with the understanding that the publisher is not engaged in rendering legal, accounting, or other professional service. If legal advice or other expert assistance is required, the services of a competent professional person should be sought." (From a Declaration of Principles jointly adopted by a Committee of the American Bar Association and a Committee of Publishers and Associations.)

Issue: Vol. 2, No. 3 ISBN: 0-89443-431-4
ISSN: 0271-8294
Printed in the United States of America.

Contents

Language Disorders of Hearing-Impaired Children

- vi   **Letters to the editor**
- vii   **From the editor**
- viii   **R. Curtis Whitesel: In Memoriam**
- ix   **Foreword**
- 1   **After early identification: next steps for language intervention for very young severely hearing-impaired children**
Janelle M. Spear and Sanford E. Gerber
- 8   **Early intervention and development of communication skills for deaf children using an auditory–verbal approach**
Ellen A. Rhoades
- 17   **Overcoming linguistic limitations of hearing-impaired children through teaching written language**
Danny D. Steinberg
- 29   **Amplification: tool for language skills**
Mark Ross
- 46   **Language assessment protocols for hearing-impaired students**
Diane Brackett
- 57   **Language intervention for hearing-impaired children from linguistically and culturally diverse backgrounds**
Joseph E. Fischgrund
- 67   **Assessing language in young deaf adults**
Gerard G. Walter and C. Tane Akamatsu
- 76   **Societal forces influencing the roles of speech–language pathologists, audiologists, and teachers of the deaf**
E. Harris Nober
- 88   **Notices**

Editorial board

Editor
Katharine G. Butler, PhD
Director
Division of Special Education
 & Rehabilitation
Syracuse University
Syracuse, New York

Board

James L. Aten, PhD
Chief, Audiology and Speech
 Pathology Service
Department of Audiology and
 Speech Pathology
Long Beach Veterans Administration
 Medical Center
Long Beach, California

Jack W. Birch, PhD
Professor
School of Education
University of Pittsburgh
Pittsburgh, Pennsylvania

Roger Brown, PhD
John Lindsley Professor of Psychology
Department of Psychology and
 Social Relations
Harvard University
Cambridge, Massachusetts

Robert C. Calfee, PhD
1981–1982 Fellow
Center for Advanced Study
 in the Behavioral Sciences
School of Education
Stanford University
Stanford, California

Sara E. Conlon, PhD
Executive Director
Alexander Graham Bell Association
 for the Deaf, Inc.
Washington, D.C.

Leo E. Connor, EdD
Executive Director
Lexington School for the Deaf
Jackson Heights, New York

Richard J. Dowling, MS, JD
Executive Director
American Society of Allied
 Health Professions
Washington, D.C.

Drake D. Duane, MD
Associate Professor of Neurology
Mayo Medical School
Mayo Clinic/Foundation
Rochester, Minnesota

Sylvia Farnham-Diggory, PhD
H. Rodney Sharp Professor
Department of Educational Studies
 and Psychology
University of Delaware
Newark, Delaware

Diane Frost
Committee Member
Association for Children and Adults with
 Learning Disabilities
Pittsburgh, Pennsylvania

Ronald Goldman, PhD
Professor
Department of Biocommunication
Center for Developmental and
 Learning Disorders
University of Alabama in Birmingham
Birmingham, Alabama

William C. Healey, PhD
Professor
Department of Special Education
Adjunct Professor
Department of Speech and Hearing
 Sciences
University of Arizona
Tucson, Arizona

David Ingram, PhD
Associate Professor
Department of Linguistics
University of British Columbia
Vancouver, British Columbia

Doris J. Johnson, PhD
Head, Program in Learning
 Disabilities
Professor of Learning Disabilities
Learning Disabilities Center
Northwestern University
Evanston, Illinois

James F. Kavanagh, PhD
Associate Director
Center for Research for Mothers and
 Children
National Institute of Child Health
 and Human Development
National Institutes of Health
Bethesda, Maryland

Merlin J. Mecham, PhD
Professor of Speech Pathology
Department of Communication
University of Utah
Salt Lake City, Utah

Rita C. Naremore, PhD
Chairperson
Department of Speech and Hearing
 Sciences
Indiana University
Bloomington, Indiana

Bruce Porch, PhD
Speech Pathologist
Veterans Administration
 Medical Center
Albuquerque, New Mexico

Sylvia O. Richardson, MA, MD
Formerly Associate Professor of
 Pediatrics
University of Cincinnati College of Medicine
Distinguished Professor of Communicology
Clinical Professor of Pediatrics
University of South Florida
Tampa, Florida

Jane A. Rieke, MA
Coordinator, Communication Programs
Experimental Education Unit
Child Development and Mental
 Retardation Center
University of Washington
Seattle, Washington

Joseph G. Sheehan, PhD
Professor of Psychology
University of California
Los Angeles, California

Richard L. Schiefelbusch, PhD
Director
Bureau of Child Research & Kansas
 Center for Mental Retardation and
 Human Development
University of Kansas
Lawrence, Kansas

Catherine E. Snow, PhD
Visiting Associate Professor
Graduate School of Education
Harvard University
Cambridge, Massachusetts

Joel Stark, PhD
Professor and Director
Speech and Hearing Center
Department of Communication Arts
 and Sciences
Queens College of the City University
 of New York
Flushing, New York

David A. Stumpf, MD, PhD
Director of Pediatric Neurology
Associate Professor of Pediatrics
 and Neurology
University of Colorado Health
 Sciences Center
Denver, Colorado

Geraldine P. Wallach, PhD
Associate Professor
Department of Communication
 Disorders
Emerson College
Boston, Massachusetts

Joanna P. Williams, PhD
Professor of Psychology and
 Education
Department of Psychology
Teachers College, Columbia
 University
New York, New York

Rhonda S. Work, MA
Consultant, Speech and
  Language Impaired
Bureau of Education for
  Exceptional Students
Florida Department of
  Education
Tallahassee, Florida

David E. Yoder, PhD
Walker-Bascom Professor
Department of Communicative
  Disorders
University of Wisconsin—Madison
Madison, Wisconsin

Naomi Zigmond, PhD
Professor
Director of Special Education Program
School of Education
Research Associate
Learning Research and Development
  Center
University of Pittsburgh
Pittsburgh, Pennsylvania

Letters to the editor

All letters to the editor should be addressed to Editor, TLD, Aspen Systems Corporation, 1600 Research Boulevard, Rockville, MD 20850. Unless otherwise stated, we assume that letters addressed to the editor are intended for publication with your name and affiliation. As many letters as possible will be published. When space is limited and we cannot publish all letters received, we will select letters reflecting the range of opinions and ideas received. If a letter merits a response from an author or the editor, we will obtain a reply and publish both letters.

From the editor

Not thou, not thou—'tis we
Are deaf, are dumb, are blind.
Edmund C. Stedman
Helen Keller, Stanza 4
Circa 1833–1908

Helen Keller represents to many of us the heights that can be attained by an individual suffering from the dual handicaps of deafness and blindness. Stedman's quote captures a sense of the world's admiration for this extraordinary woman, but he fails to differentiate between the consequences of the two handicaps. However, Helen Keller is reported to have commented on the impact of hearing impairment when she said, "I am just as deaf as I am blind. The problems of deafness are deeper and more complex, if not more important than those of blindness. Deafness is a much worse misfortune. For it means the loss of the most vital stimulus—the sound of the voice that brings language, sets thoughts astir and keep us in the company of man" (S. Conlon, Executive Director, Alexander Graham Bell Association for the Deaf, personal communication, January 13, 1982).

Indeed, it is the depth and complexity of language disorders resulting from hearing impairment that has challenged and frustrated teachers of the deaf, speech–language pathologists, and audiologists over time. Major areas of disagreement regarding the best approach(es) to habilitation of the hearing impaired have spanned the past century. But as Brill (1974) noted, there *is* agreement among educators that "the major handicapping condition of deafness is lack of communication" (p. 189). This theme is often repeated in the literature, as is a second theme that deals with the early speech and language training of infants and toddlers (Clarke & Rogers, 1981; Miller, 1981).

Dr. Linda Nober, Issue Editor, has provided a review of what is and a preview of what may be, judiciously blending research and practice. There is a sense of urgency in this issue, as well there might be. There is some evidence that early deafness has become relatively as well as actually more prevalent over the past four decades (Schein & Delk, 1974). Thus, we may anticipate an increasing need for thoughtful and appropriate speech and language training, habilitation, and education for the hearing impaired.

Long ago, Helen Keller noted that "speech is the birthright of every child. It is the deaf child's one fair chance to keep in touch with his fellows" (S. Conlon, personal communication, January 13, 1982). When there is limited acoustic feedback, learning speech and language is difficult and slow. It requires much of the child; it also requires much of the teacher. The rewards to those who teach language to the hearing impaired are reflected by Helen Keller's statement that "Before my teacher came to me, I did not know that I am. I lived in a world that was a no-world" (Lash, 1980, p. 338). Teachers who work with the hearing impaired must bring an understanding of, and information about, speech and language, hearing aids and amplification, as well as curriculum modification (Davis, Shepard, Stelmachowic, & Gorga, 1981). This issue of TLD is dedicated to that proposition.

Katharine G. Butler, PhD
Editor

REFERENCES

Brill, R.G. *The education of the deaf: Administrative and professional developments.* Washington, D.C.: Gallaudet College Press, 1974.

Clarke, B.R., & Rogers, W.T. Correlates of syntatic abilities in hearing-impaired students. *Journal of Speech and Hearing Research* 1981, 24(1), 48–54.

Davis, J.M., Shepard, N.T., Stelmachowic, P.G., & Gorga, M.P. Perception of hearing impairment held by school personnel: Suggestions for in-service training development. *Language, Speech and Hearing Services in the Schools*, 1981, *12*, 168–177.

Lash, J.P. *Helen and teacher* (Radcliffe Biography Series). New York: Delacorte Press, 1980.

Miller, G.A. *Language and speech*. San Francisco: Freeman, 1981.

Schein, J.D., & Delk, T.K. *The deaf population in the United States*. Silver Spring, Md.; National Association of the Deaf, 1974.

R. Curtis Whitesel: In Memoriam

Topics in Language Disorders (TLD) exists because of the perception of a single individual. He perceived the need for a publication that would bring together those interested in language acquisition, language disorders, and language intervention. Some time ago he met with me regarding the possibility of developing a transdisciplinary journal that would be essential to professionals with those interests. He envisioned a journal that would embody the best of what is known and what yet might be. Not for "Curt" the tried and true. Not for Curt the fields well-plowed. It was the land that lay beyond that fascinated him.

TLD is now well into its second year of life, and planning for double that period has been completed. Curt was delighted with the growth of the journal and with the plans for the future. Suddenly, Curt is no longer here. Those of us who worked closely with him will miss him sorely. As Journal Editor, I would like to dedicate this issue of *Topics in Language Disorders* to a man who knew it was important, possible, and necessary to address the needs of the language disordered. During the last year of his life he interacted with more than one speech–language pathologist as he acquired a superior level of skill with esophageal speech. He came to know on most intimate terms some of the issues that the journal addresses.

I deeply regret that Curt is not here to see this issue and those that will follow. Each is a testimonial to his foresight and perseverance. My appreciation for his assistance and support remains undiminished. His contribution to our field continues.

Katharine G. Butler, PhD
—Editor

Foreword

As this issue of *Topics in Language Disorders* was being prepared, it became evident to those of us involved in the education of students with various language handicaps that we are on the threshold of an altered state of the art. In various ways, the contributors to this issue have helped shape the educational delivery system to hearing-impaired children within this country and in many other countries. The authors represent a group of professionals whose backgrounds encompass several discrete academic disciplines. They have focused their energies and talents during the past decades toward enhancing educational services to hearing-impaired children. Although current in-service and training programs involve students in different ways than those programs designed in the 1950s and 1960s, the diversity of programs designed to train professionals to work with hearing-impaired children is mirrored by the academic focus of these authors: speech–language pathology, audiology, education of the deaf, early childhood education, linguistics and special education. The complexity of language problems of hearing-impaired children requires interdisciplinary resolutions.

Several contributors have focused on the early intervention aspects of language programs for the hearing impaired. Gerber and Spear address the concept of multimodal instruction as an initiating protocol for language training, Rhoades describes a unilateral approach that relys on audition, and Steinberg documents a singular approach based on written language training. These authors represent training expertise based in speech–language pathology and audiology, education of the deaf, and linguistics, respectively.

A strong commitment to proper amplification fitting and monitoring is explained by Ross, and examples are provided that redirect the thinking of audiologists vis-à-vis children with hearing sensitivity deficiencies. Brackett helps readers to reassess the types of evaluation tools selected by teachers and clinicians. Her paper forces those service providers who find comfort and obligation within standardized assessment procedures to alter their methodology and routine.

Frishgrund presents in detail the arguments and controversies that have evolved concerning students from linguistically or culturally different backgrounds and the selection of language intervention programs for such students. Even though many professionals dedicated to education of hearing-impaired children are embroiled in the classic and fundamental arguments concerning method of language instruction, a more pressing need has evolved in many urban parts of the country regarding language instruction for non-English-speaking students.

These issues provoke reaction in readers regarding assessment of language ability for older hearing-impaired students as Walter and Akamatsu detail for us. Although the perceived dichotomy of oral English and sign language remains among professionals, these authors catalogue assessment needs within the two primary modalities of communication for the hearing impaired. The area of language usage and difficulties of mature hearing-impaired persons is often overlooked. Walter and Akamatsu provide us with specific cautions for evaluation, with implications for earlier interventions.

The totality of this field of language difficulties of the hearing impaired and the forces that impinge on the thinking, methods, and training programs of speech–language pathologists are summarized in Nober's article. He defines those societal and cultural forces within our history that have shaped and molded our mutual fields of study. Many teachers and clinicians have experienced professional school training and, therefore, have skimmed or de-emphasized those historical aspects of services to handicapped children as a study area.

When this issue of *Topics in Language Disorders* was conceptualized, our planning and organizational efforts seemed to focus on the most current aspects of knowledge about serving hearing-impaired students within regular education settings, since over 70% of the identified hearing-impaired students in this country receive their education in this setting. This choice was made due to the enormous scope of the field and our interest in providing specific information about a subgroup of hearing-impaired students many teachers and clinicians serve. Perhaps because of the extensive history of this field, and the dedication of the collected authors of this volume, the issue touches most of the pressing concerns of professionals who work with hearing-impaired individuals and their families.

We need to conceptualize a national system in which we may have to share information, expertise, and concerns about handicapped individuals within different parameters, different from those achieved under PL 94-142. The contributions of these authors have been in some part stimulated by a federalism that addresses higher education, technical education, and the upgrading of elementary and secondary education for all citizens including the hearing impaired. It is evident that those of us committed to improving services to hearing-impaired students (and other special needs students) will have to direct our energies and skills within a new structure. This collection of articles may assist us in reaching such goals without federal assistance. It may enable us to attain qualitative changes in services to the handicapped within those settings in which we serve others.

Linda W. Nober
Issue editor

After early identification: next steps for language intervention for very young severely hearing-impaired children

Janelle M. Spear, BS
Department of Speech
University of California
Santa Barbara, California

Sanford E. Gerber, PhD
Professor of Audiology
Chair, Department of Speech
University of California
Santa Barbara, California

THE ISSUE presented here has been controversial for centuries. Some of the controversy arises from a misunderstanding of the applications and principles involved. It is important to realize that hearing impairment is one of the most frequently occurring disabilities in North America today. It must be remembered that only 2% of the hearing-impaired population are truly deaf and also that congenital deafness occurs only once in about 1,200 births. This article discusses an extremely small proportion of the hearing-impaired population, the congenitally deaf, yet we consider it to be the one most interesting and most deserving of our attention and skills.

A second principle is that, with the rarest exceptions, the auditory method is always employed. We do not mean an acoupedic method that excludes all that is not auditory but only that audition should be used no matter what else is being done. Virtually every congenitally deaf infant should have one, and preferably two, hearing aids at the earliest possible age. There is no age that is too young for diagnosis and no time that is too soon to begin habilitation.

The issue of addition and subtraction was raised in a recent volume edited by Mencher and Gerber (1981). *Addition* refers to the exclusion of all methods but one from the educational procedures applied to particular deaf infants and addition or substitution of other methods later. *Subtraction*, then, is to begin with certain methods and drop some of them later. The argument presented in this article is one in favor of subtraction. Addition, in our point of view, implies failure and that the deaf infant does not have a right to be deaf. We resolve with Mencher and Gerber (1981) that as clinicians and educators it is essential "to assure—and where possible, to provide—all means which accrue to the benefit of the hearing impaired infant"— (p. 1). At the same time, we wish to ensure (as did Ling, 1981) "that, if at all possible, hearing-impaired children develop effective spoken language skills from early infancy" (p. 319).

For the past few centuries, the field of deaf education has generally been split in two distinct philosophical positions: (a) the view that all hearing-impaired children should learn language only through the "natural" oral/aural mode and (b) the belief that all available language modes (oral/aural as well as visual/motor) should be utilized. In recent years, a considerable volume of research has appeared in the area of sign language and bimodal language acquisition, yet in spite of this, comparatively little progress has been made in the attempt to come to a common agreement on this particular issue.

Both sides undoubtedly have similar long-range goals: to improve speech, listening skills, language, academic ability, and the quality of psychological well-being among severely hearing-impaired children. Similarly, there is no dispute as to whether children whose hearing impairments are in the mild to moderately severe range can function with oral/aural language alone. For children with more severe impairments, however, the question as it exists today is only a slightly modified version of the old "oral versus manual" one. Should a manual communication system be added to or substituted for an oral/aural training approach when a child fails to acquire oral language? Or does the therapist begin the child's education using a genuinely total method and subtract either the oral or manual component as it appears appropriate? The answer to this addition versus subtraction issue would be simple if definitive answers existed to the following questions: Does the use of a visual/motor system of communication (such as sign language) inhibit or preclude the simultaneous development of oral language? Does a visual/motor system of communication fulfill the requirements of a true language? Can sign language adequately meet the communicative needs of deaf individuals?

INHIBIT OR ENHANCE?

Those who advocate the addition philosophy do so on the assumption that manual communication somehow interferes or competes with the development of oral language. Ling (1976), for example, stated that "it appears highly unlikely that a child learning signs and speech can attend to both simultaneously" (p. 60). In a recent attempt to substantiate this belief, Ling (1981) cited a study by Jensema and Trybus (1978), claiming that it "showed that the use of signs among school aged children tended to replace rather than enhance speech development" (p. 321), that "subjects academic achievements were shown to be negatively correlated with sign language use but positively correlated with speech" (p. 321), and that "among the 657 children studied, those who signed most used speech least" (p. 321). Though his report on the statistical data may be reasonably accurate, his conclusions based on those data are at best overly optimistic. The authors (Jensema & Trybus, 1978) clearly emphasized that many of the variables reported that show clear relationships with speech use and sign use are also overlapping in their variance. With regard to the academic achievement findings, they stated that "while factors such as the child's hearing level and the family's income level have a large influence on the child's school achievement, variations in communication methods, specifically in the amount of speech used and amount of signs used, have little relationships with achievement scores, given the existing national variations in the quantity and quality of use of those methods" (p. 19). Furthermore, Ling was apparently misconstruing the finding that those who signed most used speech least to mean that those who signed most used speech least because of their signing. Correlation does not imply causation. It may be that those who sign most do so because they have a greater auditory deficit and/or possess fewer oral skills. In other words, it may be true (as Ling suggested) that signing inhibited the acquisition of speech, but it is at least as probable that these children preferred to sign because of their poor oral skills or oral education. The cause and effect relationship, if there is one, is not obvious. In any case, Jensema and Trybus (1978) also observed that what is true at school is not usually true at home. They noted that "there is relatively little consistency between patterns of communication used at home and in school" (p. 8). This too is not surprising, since the large majority of deaf children do not have deaf parents. Furthermore, hearing children of deaf parents are typically "native" signers, but their speech development is not impaired. Finally, of the many studies done in this area, few if any, support the notion of inhibition (e.g., Schlesinger & Meadow, 1972).

A significant number of studies have shown that a visual/motor system of communication does not interfere with, and may actually enhance, the development of academic, language, and speech-reading skills. A study by Stuckless and Birch (1966) found early manual communication to facilitate the acquisition of language in deaf students, as manifest through reading comprehension and written expression. Quigley (1969) showed that deaf children educated with both

> *It may be true that signing inhibited the acquisition of speech, but it is at least as probable that these children preferred to sign because of their poor oral skills or oral education.*

oral/aural training and a manual system (fingerspelling) performed significantly better throughout a 5-year time span on education and language tests than children taught with fewer or no use of manual supplements. Furthermore, Vernon and Koh (1971) found a group of deaf children (whose deaf parents had extremely low educational levels) who grew up in a signing environment to be superior academically and in language skills to children who had had intensive oral preschool training. Schlesinger (1978) found that deaf youngsters who were exposed to sign language exhibited their first sign earlier than hearing youngsters normally acquire their first word and that the deaf children's vocabularies were accelerated.

Other studies have demonstrated that information obtained through a visual/motor modality can enhance speech-reading skills. In experiments by Berger and Popelka (1971) and Popelka and Berger (1971), extrafacial gestures were found to enhance speech-reading performance substantially. Similarly, Schlesinger and Meadow (1972) documented an increase in spoken words with increased sign language acquisition.

The study of deaf children of deaf parents has also provided information on the effects of early and consistent use of sign language. As compared with deaf children of hearing parents, these children do better academically and psychologically (Brasel & Quigley, 1977; Brill, 1960, 1969; Meadow, 1969; Quigley & Frisina, 1961; Vernon & Koh, 1970, 1971). Why are deaf children of deaf parents superior in these respects? Since most deaf parents communicate manually with their youngsters from an early age, at least partial credit must be given to the communication mode employed. However, other factors, such as parental expectation, acceptance, and social interaction, undoubtedly contribute to this phenomenon.

One of the major concerns of those advocating the addition philosophy has been that sign language might somehow prevent the child from acquiring adequate speech. In Vernon and Koh's (1971) study, no significant differences in speech intelligibility were found between the group of deaf children who grew up in the signing environment and the children who had intensive oral preschool training. Likewise, Schlesinger and Meadow (1972) found that the knowledge of sign language in their four deaf children had not interfered with speech acquisition.

One always turns to the monumental study of Quigley (1969), in which it was found that there were no differences in the speech abilities of children taught by an oral-only method and those taught by a Rochester method (i.e., with speech and fingerspelling). As one would expect, the children taught by the Rochester method had better fingerspelling skills than those taught by a unimodal oral method, but to repeat, there were no differences in their own oral skills. Ling (1981) observed that there is no evidence that early use of manual skills enhances speech; the opposite is also true. These findings suggest that the notion of inhibition is false. That is, the use of a visual/motor system of communication, such as sign language or fingerspelling, apparently does not inhibit or preclude the development of speech, language, and related skills.

BUT IS IT LANGUAGE?

The question of whether sign language can adequately meet the communicative needs of deaf individuals has been a matter of concern to educators for many decades. One of the arguments has been that sign language is too limited or lacking in complexity. Those unfamiliar with American Sign Language (ASL) question its ability to represent symbolic concepts and argue against its highly iconic nature. ASL has also been criticized as being ungrammatical, hence, a poor substitute for English. Though a considerable amount of systematic research needs to be done in this area, it appears that sign language meets the criteria necessary for language and can adequately serve the needs of those who are denied access to unobscured oral language.

ASL, the sign system used by most deaf American adults, has been shown to be a language with its own morphology, syntax, and semantics (Bellugi & Klima, 1978). Markowicz (1980) explains that the myth that ASL is ungrammatical is based on the assumption that ASL must be structured exactly like English and is usually the result of sign-for-word translation of ASL into English. Though ASL has a grammar and vocabulary that are unrelated to English, it is no less a language for it. Mayberry (1978) summarized the similarities of manual communication and oral language:

1. Both sign and oral languages are created by human communities to meet their individual communicative needs.
2. Both sign and oral languages are acquired as first languages by the children of these communities.
3. Both kinds of languages are structured information codes consisting of three linguistic levels: phonetic—the pattern of the physical signal; syntactic—the relationship of the symbols; and lexical–semantic—the organization of the symbols' meanings.
4. To translate any sign or oral language into another sign or oral language, varying degrees of reorganization at each linguistic level are required.

In comparing the course of acquisition for sign and oral language, investigators have generally found more similarities than differences. Schlesinger and Meadow's (1972) study of four deaf children indicated that the milestones in sign language parallel those in spoken language acquisition. In viewing the linguistic and psychological properties of ASL, Siple (1978) found the course of language acquisition to be strikingly similar for both ASL and oral languages. Babbling occurs at approximately 6 months of age for both deaf and normal hearing youngsters—in a gesturing modality for the former and verbally for the latter. At about 1 year, children begin to produce one-word utterances, whereas at the same age, deaf children in a sign environment begin to produce single signs. In addition, at about 18 to 24 months, normal hearing children are beginning to construct two-word strings, and deaf children are similarly forming two-sign strings (Siple, 1978). Collins-Ahlgren (1975) noted the same type of overgeneralization patterns seen in the development of our spoken language. For instance, the sign for *dog* was used initially to represent all animals, the sign for *mother* referred to a caretaking person of either sex, and *water* meant a drink of any kind. Eventually the terms narrowed in their intended referents.

As mentioned previously, ASL has been criticized by some as being highly iconic and concrete. Markowicz (1980) and Siple (1978) demonstrated that this belief is not substantiated by linguistic analysis and observation of ASL. As they pointed out, ASL includes signs for abstract concepts, such as love, belief, hope, and wisdom. Furthermore, sign language is used regularly to conduct religious services for deaf congregations and an unlimited number of other situations requiring all of the nuances and abstractions handled by spoken English. Given the preceding data, we stress with Gerber and Prutting (1981) that "arguments in favor or against the use of sign language in the education of deaf children should not include the linguistic status of the language, as value judgments are no longer credible" (p. 339). Furthermore, they insisted that the deaf should be bilingual.

A TOTAL APPROACH

In light of findings discussed here, it is difficult to see how any early management program but a total one could be justified for those children who are truly deaf. Bess and McConnell (1981) reminded us that such children depend primarily on vision for their reception of language symbols, by via manual message with or without speech reading. Hence, maximum achievement is accomplished by introduction of such methods at the earliest possible age.

Some criticism has arisen due to the fact that many current deaf education programs mislabel themselves as "total" and fail to provide a total service. Pahz and Pahz (1978) describe total communication as incorporating the combined system with the oral system and everything else to put the child at the center of our attention. To be effective, a program must be designed and implemented by professionals who adhere to this philosophy.

It is apparent that the deaf child is afforded the best linguistic and communicative advantages by learning sign language at a very early age, along with intensive oral training. For those children who learn to function well without the use of signs and who do not live in a social environment where sign language is necessary, this component may be subtracted from their education. Conversely, though not as likely, there may be children whose hearing is so defective that a long-term oral training program may prove to be futile. Whether or not one of the components is subtracted, however, it is important that the deaf child have at his or her disposal all available mechanisms for communication. The hearing child is intrinsically granted all of the social, emotional, and intellectual benefits of an efficient language system. The conditions for a deaf child should not be less.

REFERENCES

Bellugi, U., & Klima, E. Structural properties of American Sign Language. In L.S. Liben (Ed.), *Deaf children: Developmental perspectives*. New York: Academic Press, 1978.

Berger, K., & Popelka, G. Extra-facial gestures in relation to speechreading. *Journal of Communication Disorders*, 1971, 3, 302–308.

Bess, F.H., & McConnell, F.E. *Audiology, education, and the hearing impaired child*. St. Louis, Mo.: Mosby, 1981.

Brasel, K., & Quigley, S. Influence of certain language and communication environments in early childhood on the development of language in deaf individuals. *Journal of Speech and Hearing Research*, 1977, 20, 95–107.

Brill, R.G. A study in adjustment of three groups of deaf children. *Exceptional Children*, 1960, 26, 464–466.

Brill, R.G. The superior I.Q.'s of deaf children of deaf parents. *The California Palms*, 1969, 1–4.

Collins-Ahlgren, M. Language development of two deaf children. *American Annals of the Deaf*, 1975, 120, 524–539.

Gerber, S.E., & Prutting, C.A. Bilingualism: An environment for the deaf infant. In G.T. Mencher & S.E. Gerber (Eds.) *Early management of hearing loss*. New York: Grune & Stratton, 1981.

Jensema, C., & Trybus, R. *Communication patterns and educational achievements of hearing impaired students* (Series T, Number 2). Washington, D.C.: Office of Demographic Studies, Gallaudet College, 1978.

Ling, D. *Speech and the hearing-impaired child: Theory and practice*. Washington, D.C.: A.G. Bell, 1976.

Ling, D. Early speech development. In G.T. Mencher & S.E. Gerber (Eds.), *Early management of hearing loss*. New York: Grune & Stratton, 1981.

Markowicz, H. Myths about American Sign Language. In H. Lane & F. Grosjean (Eds.), *Recent perspectives on American Sign Language*. Hillsdale, N.J.: Erlbaum, 1980.

Mayberry, R. Manual communication. In H. Davis & S.R. Silverman (Eds.), *Hearing and deafness* (4th ed.). New York: Holt, Rinehart & Winston, 1978.

Meadow, K.P. Self image, family climate, and deafness. *Social Forces*, 1969, 47, 428–438.

Mencher, G.T., & Gerber, S.E. (Eds.). *Early management of hearing loss*. New York: Grune & Stratton, 1981.

Pahz, J., & Pahz, C. *Total communication: The meaning behind the movement to expand educational opportunities for deaf children*. Springfield, Ill.: Charles C Thomas, 1978.

Popelka, G., & Berger, K. Gestures and visual speech reception. *American Annals of the Deaf*, 1971, 116, 434–436.

Quigley, S. *The influence of fingerspelling on the development of language communication and educational achievement in deaf children*. Urbana: University of Illinois, Institute for Research on Exceptional Children, 1969.

Quigley, S., & Frisina, D.R. Institutionalization and psycho-educational development of deaf children. *Council for Exceptional Children Research Monograph*, 1961, 3.

Schlesinger, H. The acquisition of signed and spoken language. In L.S. Liben (Ed.), *Deaf children: Developmental perspectives*. New York: Academic Press, 1978.

Schlesinger, H., & Meadow, K. *Sound and sign: Childhood deafness and mental health*. Berkeley: University of California Press, 1972.

Siple, P. Linguistic and psychological properties of American Sign Language: An overview. In P. Siple (Ed.), *Understanding language through sign language research*. New York: Academic Press, 1978.

Stuckless, E.R., & Birch, J.W. The influence of early manual communication on the linguistic development of deaf children. *American Annals of the Deaf*, 1966, 111, 452–504.

Vernon, M., & Koh, S.D. Early manual communication and deaf children's achievement. *American Annals of the Deaf*, 1970, 115, 527–536.

Vernon, M., & Koh, S.D. Effects of oral preschool compared to early manual communication on education and communication in deaf children. *American Annals of the Deaf*, 1971, 116, 569–574.

Early intervention and development of communication skills for deaf children using an auditory–verbal approach

Ellen A. Rhoades, EdS
Director
Auditory Educational Clinic
Atlanta, Georgia

In his acceptance speech after receiving the Wallin Award from the Council for Exceptional Children, Lloyd M. Dunn (1980) asserted:

I implore us as a group to become more scholarly.... Often we are too satisfied with our own approaches and too critical of those used by others. In my view, this is a sign that our field is made up of fragmented splinter groups of technicians, rather than of comprehensively trained scholars.... First, in education of the deaf, there is still a wide schism between the oralists and manualists. I know. I recently tried to get a balanced chapter on education of the deaf written, and failed. (pp. 150–151)

The oral–manual controversy, more than 150 years old, continues, albeit under the present-day rubric of aural–oral advocates versus the total communication of simultaneous advocates. Oralists argue that speech is necessary for communication within our society. Manualists argue that speech is secondary to language; that speech reading as the sole means of learn-

0271-8294/82/0023-0008$2.00
© 1982 Aspen Systems Corporation

ing language is, at best, difficult; and that without language the deaf are prevented from communicating even within a deaf subculture, becoming socially, linguistically, academically, and vocationally disadvantaged. Both arguments appear valid (Ling, 1975). It would be preferable to have deaf children develop readily intelligible speech as well as linguistic competence. For the majority of deaf children who learn through the visual modality, however, this does not appear to be the case (Furth, 1966).

A commonality of both of these approaches is that of a multisensory outlook on educating deaf children, predicated on the proposition that language skills should be taught through as many sensory modalities as possible. Whether through speech reading, sign language, finger spelling, hand cues, the printed symbol, or any combination thereof, visual input is generally the predominant means of teaching communication skills. Other sensory avenues (audition, taction, kinesthetics) are explored and developed in these multisensory approaches for the purpose of assisting in the child's visually oriented speech and language development. Moreover, these multisensory approaches assume that the child with severe or profound hearing loss is deaf and therefore cannot efficiently process language primarily through the auditory channel.

THEORETICAL ANTECEDENTS OF THE AUDITORY-VERBAL APPROACH

Hearing impairment

Children labeled as deaf are those with severe to profound hearing losses without the use of amplification; they demonstrate unaided hearing thresholds of 91 dB or worse in the speech range. Such an audiometric definition of deafness is usually accompanied by an educational definition that states the need for classes or schools for the deaf (e.g., Silverman, 1963).

However, the fact that at least 95% of these deaf children have some usable residual hearing must not be overlooked (Ling & Ling, 1978). Given the current technology of hearing aids, these children are capable of hearing conversational levels of speech. It is thus possible that deaf children can function as hard-of-hearing children, providing they have appropriate amplification. Aided hearing thresholds then appear more important for consideration of a child's educational classification (Pollack, 1970). Perhaps it is an injustice to label these children as deaf rather than as hearing impaired. This is not to deny their deafness, but to prevent the foreordaining of their level of functional hearing.

Levels of expectation

Research bears out the notion of the self-fulfilling prophecy (Jones, 1977). When people perceive an individual to be deaf, they tend to noticeably adjust their interactional patterns with that individual, since our expectations for that individual's communication skills tend to be altered to some degree. It logically appears to follow that their expectations of a hard-of-hearing child would differ from those of a deaf child, since their interactional pattern adjustments would not warrant as much modification.

Sensory modality

The research also indicates that one does not attend equally well to competing visual and auditory stimulation; one can attend to selected portions of each sensory input but not to all of each (Stewart, Pollack, & Downs, 1964). Therefore, language, if learned primarily through the unimpaired visual channel, is likely to be acquired at the expense of auditory development. To optimally develop the child's remaining hearing for learning language, it is necessary to focus on that one sensory modality without competing visual stimuli.

Developmental perspective

Although children develop at different rates, they tend to develop in a sequential, hierarchical manner. Complex speech, language, and listening skills are based on essential processes of development, such as turn-taking patterns (Gratch, 1979). Vocalizations and babbling emerge into speech and connected language; auditory development progresses from awareness of sound to discrimination of speech sounds. It can be assumed, then, that children would benefit from passing through the milestones in developmental stages of speech and language.

Parental importance

Evidence indicates that parents are the major influence in their children's lives from infancy through preschool years. Parents are their child's most natural reinforcing agents as well as their child's primary and most effective teachers (Gordon, Greenwood, Ware, & Olmstead, 1974). The role of audition is considered important in achieving normal parent–infant interaction (Condon & Sander, 1974). Such parent–child interactions lay the groundwork for the child's linguistic competence (Bateson, 1975). Thus, the parents' role in the child's language development is of great importance (Anderson, Vietze, & Dokecki, 1977). Moreover, direct parent–child verbal interaction is amenable to guidance and improvement (Jason, 1977; Price, 1977).

Normal models of speech and language

We speak as we hear, and children will imitate what they hear. Because they are learning to hear, they need to be exposed to normal speech and language models. There appears to be a logical interplay between selective auditory sensitivity and ease of production of speech sounds (Northern & Downs, 1978). Moreover, the techniques of modeling, expectation, expansion, imitation, and parallel talk appear to facilitate language construction (Cazden, 1972). Hearing-impaired children can benefit from language models provided by their parents and hearing peers, who appropriately adjust their linguistic levels to the development level of their listener (Guralnick & Paul-Brown, 1977).

Importance of early years

The early childhood years are formative years for learning auditory–verbal communication skills. The notion of critical periods is paramount to optimal linguistic and auditory development prior to 3 years of age (Eisenberg, 1976).

Amplification

More often than not, it seems that children who wear hearing aids appear to be using ineffective or inconsistent amplification (Gaeth & Lounsbury, 1966; Ross, 1977; Zink, 1972). Those not receiving consistent and systematic audiological management make poor use of their residual hearing (Hanners, 1973). The literature suggests that lack of early and systematic auditory stimulation causes neurological deterioration through disease (Barnet, Griffiths, & Wedenberg, 1965; Koegel & Felsenfeld, 1977).

The literature suggests that lack of early and systematic auditory stimulation causes neurological deterioration through disease.

PREMISES OF THE THIRD WAY

Certain premises are considered necessary components for any auditory–verbal education to be optimally effective so that deaf children can become functionally listening individuals. Based on the above, requisite principles (Beebe, 1978; Pollack, 1970) of the auditory–verbal approach can be summarized as

- early identification and referral, including the need for complete and ongoing audiological evaluations at the earliest possible age, preferably during infancy
- early, effective amplification, which should be consistent and preferably binaural; hearing aids fitted on the child as soon as diagnoses are made by otologists and audiologists, worn during all waking hours, and monitored daily
- early, intensive, and individualized auditory activities designed to develop a listening function, with the child not being taught to speech read
- early, active family involvement whereby parents participate in daily listening activities
- early mainstreaming, which prevents placement of the child in a special preschool class for the deaf
- early language development from a normal developmental perspective, which involves a generally nonanalytical or natural approach, and linguistic stimulation within meaningful context of the child's daily experiences and interests
- early speech development through an auditory feedback mechanism designed to elicit imitation and babbling from the child.

DEVELOPMENT OF AUDITORY-VERBAL SKILLS

The child needs to become aware of sound stimuli and to develop a selective focus for audiological awareness, or a perceptual set. Attention to a variety of sounds is a prelude to localizing the source of these sounds (sound–object association), recognizing their meaning, reacting appropriately to them, and imitating or using such sounds. As Pollack (1970) emphasizes, the core of these listening activities includes vocal play, music, noisemakers, other environmental sounds, prespeech or prelinguistic activities such as blowing, and speech/language. As the child becomes increasingly aware of sounds, experiences are provided to encourage distance hearing, the localization of sounds, speech-sound discriminations, and gradual development of auditory memory span, voice control, speech, and language production.

Once a listening function has been developed, children can use visual cues to supplement the auditory cues to a greater degree. They become multisensory and integrate sensory stimuli in a natural way.

THE RIPPLE EFFECT

The auditory–verbal approach, influenced by European thought (Ewing, 1957; Huizing, 1959; Whetnall & Fry, 1954) has been in existence in the United States since the 1940s. The Acoupedic Program at Porter Memorial Hospital in Denver, Colorado, and the Unisensory Program at the Helen Beebe Speech and Hearing Center in Easton, Pennsylvania, are two such pioneer programs. In 1978, the International Committee on Auditory–Verbal Communication was established to demonstrate and disseminate this approach. Adopted as a special standing committee in 1980 by the Alexander Graham Bell Association for the Deaf, this Committee consists of educators, physicians, audiologists, and parents who, through their expertise, endeavor to integrate hearing into the child's total personality. The UNIsensory Project, resulting from their efforts, is part of the First Chance Network funded by the Office of Special Education's Handicapped Children's Early Education Programs. As a demonstration model program, its goal is threefold: (a) to provide an effective, comprehensive auditory–verbal approach to education for young children with severe or profound hearing losses; (b) to demonstrate that so-called deaf children can learn to hear and function as hard-of-hearing individuals and that their parents can undertake the primary responsibility for teaching them in their own home; and (c) to disseminate such a model that is both practical and cost-effective, which can be successfully replicated by other individuals or agencies serving hearing-impaired children.

UNISENSORY PROJECT SERVICES

The UNIsensory Project is a parent-oriented program serving hearing-impaired children from birth through 6 years of age in 25 counties surrounding Atlanta. Staff members function as parent advisors and demonstration therapists rather than as teachers or audiologists per se. All parents, after selecting this program as their educational option, sign an educational agreement in which they agree to undertake full responsibility for their child's program and progress based on demonstration of the child's unaided hearing loss as being the primary handicapping condition.

Parent–child focus

Delivery of parent–child services is both center and home based. Home visits by the staff involve observations of routine parent–infant verbal and nonverbal interactions, also including the quality of socioemotional relationships. Home visits are arranged weekly for infants up to 12 months of age. By the time children are 2 years old, home visits are conducted annually, with parents and children attending weekly on-site demonstration-therapy listening sessions.

All parents first participate in an orientation period, which involves individual meetings with the parent advisor for 1 hour each week over a 2-month period. They are provided with information that enables them to understand residual hearing, the care and maintenance of hearing aids, audiological evaluations and interpretations, causes of hearing loss, anatomy of the ear, and basic terminology used by staff members and other professionals in related fields—all reinforced with a great deal of printed information for inclusion in their handbook. Consequently, parents are able to intelligently ask and answer questions in their future dealings with other professionals.

After completing their orientation period, parents meet individually with the parent advisor on a monthly basis for at least 1 hour. The advisor reviews the children's overall progress, responds to the parents' questions and concerns, and provides the parents with additional information in normal child development and whatever else might be appropriate. Group meetings and workshops for all parents are also provided once each month.

Preschool

By at least 2 years of age, all enrolled children are required to be placed in regular preschool programs with normal hearing peers. However, some children are placed in preschool programs at an earlier age if both parents work outside of their home. Staff members evaluate preschool programs in neighborhoods specified by parents, and choices are given to parents as to those that would best serve the child's needs, with preferences for those preschool programs that would be cooperative in working with the project staff. Selection of a neighborhood preschool program is then based on a joint decision of parents and staff members.

Initially, a staff member and the parents meet with the preschool director and the teacher for an orientation session to discuss minimal care and use of hearing aids as well as objectives for that child's communicative skill development. The stage is then set for a mutually beneficial and cooperative relationship when suggestions are solicited from the preschool director and teacher.

A staff member visits each child in the preschool classroom for $1/2$ day each month until the child achieves either age-appropriate verbal skills or a verbal developmental age of 4 years. The staff member observes the child in relation to peers and teacher and the carry-over of the child's communication skills into the classroom. Immediately following each observation, the staff member convenes privately with the teacher to give viewpoints and to solicit information. Preschool teachers then assist advisor therapists in the annual formal assessment of the child.

Audiologists

Comprehensive audiological management services are initiated immediately

> *Preschool teachers acquire a basic working knowledge of hearing aids so they can troubleshoot minor difficulties occurring in the classroom.*

on enrollment in this project during the orientation period. Periodic otological checkups are strongly urged. Parents learn how to monitor their child's hearing aids daily. Preschool teachers acquire a basic working knowledge of hearing aids so they can troubleshoot minor difficulties that occur in the classroom.

Project staff members follow up on audiological evaluations by (a) accompanying parent and child on their periodic visits to audiologists, particularly in the first year or so, until the child is wearing optimal amplification and responds consistently and appropriately in sound conditioning tasks; (b) discussing all audiological evaluation results with parents to be sure they understand the aided and unaided audiograms; (c) informing parents of all follow-up contacts staff members have had with their audiologists and hearing aid dealers while acting as liaison between all involved parties; (d) providing weekly electroacoustic monitoring of hearing aids and, if necessary, weekly tympanometry, making earmold impressions, and earmolding cleanings; and (e) monitoring the child's aided audiological performance with a quick five-phoneme test at the outset of every demonstration therapy session.

Finally, biannual workshops are provided for all audiologists in 25 counties to inform them of the project's progress, to provide ongoing inservice, and to strive for cooperation between them as to optimal audiological management.

Child assessment

All formal assessment instruments are standardized on a nonhandicapped population, since the hearing-impaired child's progress is used relative to normal child development. The planning, implementation, and evaluation processes for each child are based on normal developmental levels; hearing age (length of time child has been aided) and chronological age are always considered. In addition to determining the child's general level of communication and overall development, five basic areas of communication skills are assessed with the assistance of parents, preschool teachers, and audiologists:

- listening skills
- auditory memory skills
- receptive language skills
- expressive language skills
- speech proficiency.

Assessment instruments are formal and informal, formative and summative. They include the parent diary; staff-made checklists and rating scales; videotapes and audiotapes; and standardized tools, such as selected subtests of the Illinois Test of Psycholinguistic Abilities, the Sequenced Inventory of Communication Development, the Alpern-Boll Developmental Profile II, the Peabody Picture Vocabulary Test–Revised, and Caldwell's HOME Inventory.

THE FUTURE

Upon completion of this 3-year demonstration model project, data will be statistically analyzed and reported. However, the sample size will be small, and unfortunately, longitudinal data cannot be extracted. A need remains for the network of auditory–verbal programs to combine their data and yield further empirical evidence. This is a research goal of the International Committee on Auditory–Verbal Communication.

It is best to continue offering the auditory–verbal approach as one of several educational options available for hearing-impaired children. Because of the frequently debilitating consequences of deafness, varied educational approaches in learning effective communication skills are necessary so that children may attain their rightful places in society. It must be recognized that diversity is healthy, and the approach must be fitted to the child. As long as an attempt to claim one approach as being right for all children exists, a great disservice is done to future hearing-impaired citizens.

REFERENCES

Anderson, B. J., Vietze, P., & Dokecki, P. R. Reciprocity in vocal interactions of mothers and infants. *Child Development*, 1977, *48*, 1676–1681.

Barnet, A., Griffiths, C., & Wedenberg, E. The young deaf child: Identification and management. *Acta Otolaryngologica*, 1965, *43*, 210–215. (Supplement 206)

Bateson, M. C. Mother–infant exchanges: The epigenesis of conversational interaction. *Annals of the New York Academy of Sciences*, 1975, *263*, 101–113.

Beebe, H. H. Deaf children can learn to hear. *Journal of Communication Disorders*, 1978, *11*, 193–200.

Cazden, C. B. Suggestions from studies of early language acquisition. In C. B. Cazden (Ed.), *Language in early childhood education*. Washington, D.C.: National Association for the Education of Young Children, 1972.

Condon, W. S., & Sander, L. W. Neonate movement is synchronized with adult speech: Interactional participation and language acquisition. *Science*, 1974, *183*, 99–101.

Dunn, L. N. Lloyd M. Dunn receives Wallin Award (Bulletin). *Exceptional Children*, 1980, *47*, 149–151.

Eisenberg, R. B. *Auditory competence in early life*. Baltimore, Md.: University Park Press, 1976.

Ewing, A. W. G. (Ed.) *Educational guidance and the deaf child*. Washington, D.C.: Volta Bureau, 1957.

Furth, H. *Thinking without language: Psychological implications of deafness*. New York: Free Press, 1966.

Gaeth, J. H., & Lounsbury, E. Hearing aids and children in elementary schools. *Journal of Speech and Hearing Disorders*, 1966, *31*, 283–289.

Gordon, I. J., Greenwood, G. E., Ware, W. B., & Olmstead, P. P. *The Florida Parent Education Follow Through Program*. Gainesville: University of Florida, Institute for Development of Human Resources, 1974.

Gratch, G. The development of thought and language in infancy. In J. P. Osofsky (Ed.), *Handbook of infant development*. New York: Wiley, 1979.

Guralnick, M. J., & Paul-Brown, D. The nature of verbal interactions among handicapped and non-handicapped preschool children. *Child Development*, 1977, *48*, 254–256.

Hanners, B. *The role of audiological management in the development of language by severely hearing impaired children*. Paper presented at the meeting of the Academy of Rehabilitation Audiology, Detroit, Michigan, 1973.

Huizing, H. Deaf-mutism—Modern trends in treatment and prevention. *Advances in Oto-Rhino-Laryngology*, 1959, *15*, 74.

Jason, L. A. Modifying parent–child interactions in a disadvantaged family. *Journal of Clinical Child Psychology*, 1977, *6*, 38–40.

Jones, R. A. *Self-fulfilling prophecies: Social, psychological, and physiological effects of expectancies*. New York: Wiley, 1977.

Koegel, R. L., & Felsenfeld, S. Critical ages in hearing. In S. Gerber (Ed.), *Audiometry in infancy*. New York: Grune & Stratton, 1977.

Ling, D. Recent developments affecting the education of hearing impaired children. *Public Health Reviews*, 1975, *4*, 117–152.

Ling, D., & Ling, A. H. *Aural habilitation: The foundations of verbal learning in hearing impaired children*. Washington, D.C.: Alexander Graham Bell Association for the Deaf, 1978.

Northern, J. L., & Downs, M. P. *Hearing in children*. Baltimore, Md.: Williams & Wilkins, 1978.

Pollack, D. *Education audiology for the limited hearing infant*. Springfield, Ill.: Charles C Thomas, 1970.

Price, G. M. *Factors influencing reciprocity in early*

mother–infant interaction. Paper presented at the meeting of the Society for Research in Child Development, New Orleans, Louisiana, 1977.

Ross, M. Definitions and descriptions. In J. Davis (Ed.), *Our forgotten children: Hard-of-hearing pupils in the schools* (National Support Systems Project). Minneapolis: University of Minnesota, 1977.

Silverman, S. R. The education of children with hearing impairments. *Journal of Pediatrics*, 1963, *62*, 254–260.

Stewart, J. L., Pollack, D., & Downs, M. P. A unisensory program for the limited hearing child. *ASHA*, 1964, *6*, 151–154.

Whetnall, E., & Fry, D. B. The auditory approach in the training of deaf children. *Lancet*, 1954, *1*, 106.

Zink, G. D. Hearing aids children wear: A longitudinal study of performance. *Volta Review*, 1972, *74*, 41–51.

Overcoming linguistic limitations of hearing-impaired children through teaching written language

Danny D. Steinberg, PhD
Department of English as a Second
  Language
University of Hawaii
Honolulu, Hawaii

RESEARCH SHOWS that the average reading level of hearing-impaired persons graduating from high school does not exceed that of normal hearing children in Grades 4 or 5 of elementary school. (For studies in America, see Furth, 1966, 1971; Lane & Baker, 1974; Wrightstone, Aronow, & Moskowitz, 1963.) Given that a portion of the hearing-impaired population has problems in acquiring literacy through the mediation of speech and sign, it is proposed that such knowledge be acquired through the direct learning of written language. The essential idea is that the basic written forms of an ordinary speech-based language such as English (e.g., its words, phrases, and sentences) are acquired initially through a direct association with objects, events, and situations in the environment. Thus, just as hearing children learn language by associating the speech sounds that they hear with environmental experiences, hearing-impaired children learn language in a similar way, but through an association of

0271-8294/82/0023-0017$2.00
© 1982 Aspen Systems Corporation

written forms with environmental experiences. As a result, hearing-impaired children acquire essentially the same vocabulary and syntax of speech-based language as hearing children because, as linguists have long noted, in a written language such as English, virtually all of the basic vocabulary and syntactic structures that appear in speech also appear in writing (e.g., subject–verb–object relations, passivation, relative clause formation, and negation).

This is not to say that there are no differences in speech and writing. There are. However, it should be observed that insofar as syntax is concerned, the differences are not great and are often more quantitative than qualitative in nature. Thus, for example, passives tend to occur more in expository writing than in speech, and sentences end with prepositions more often in speech than in writing. Essentially, however, one basic grammar underlies both mediums of expression. Because virtually any proposition or idea that can be expressed in speech can be expressed in writing, in that sense written language can be regarded as a complete language. Its main difference with speech concerns the physical means of transmission—writing involves light, whereas speech involves sound.

In teaching written language directly, six important advantages for the hearing impaired and their education may be noted:

1. The learning medium is appropriate. Perception of written stimuli depends on vision, a medium in which the normal hearing impaired have a full capability. Language can be acquired without any special obstacle on the basis of the visual medium.

2. Written language acquisition can facilitate speech. By learning written language, the syntax and vocabulary that underlie speech are also learned. Acquisition of such knowledge reduces the burden of oral instruction.

3. Written language knowledge need not be acquired by instructors. Parents and teachers of the hearing impaired do not have to learn the written language in order to teach it, since most already know it. Only instructional methods and techniques have to be acquired.

4. Instruction can begin early. Parents of hearing-impaired children can teach their children written language at home during the children's most formative years. Children as young as 1 year old can be exposed to written language in a natural way in the supportive comfort of their own home.

5. All hearing-impaired children can benefit. Effort devoted to teaching language is not wasted. All children are able to benefit from it, since whatever is learned improves their level of literacy.

6. Written language acquisition is compatible with other approaches. Written language can be taught in conjunction with other approaches, such as oral or sign, without any injury to the integrity of those approaches. One might note, in this regard, that the John Tracy Clinic of Los Angeles is experimenting with the written

language teaching program advocated here in addition to their regular oral education.

RELATED RESEARCH

Actually, the ideas proposed above are by no means new. Alexander Graham Bell (1883) taught written language to a 5-year-old deaf boy for 2 years with some success. Bell agreed with the view advocated by Dalgarno (1680/1971) 200 years before that reading and writing can be taught directly to the hearing impaired without the means of speech. Bell (1883) stated, "I believe that George Dalgarno . . . has given us the true principle to work upon when he asserts that *a deaf person should be taught to read and write in as nearly as possible the same way that young ones are taught to speak and understand their mother tongue*. We should talk to the deaf child just as we do to the hearing one, with the exception that words are to be addressed to his eye instead of his ear" (p. 126).

Since the early part of this century, there has been little interest in the teaching of written language. In the past decade, however, Lenneberg (1972) and, apparently, Lado (1976) have suggested its adoption. Some oral-oriented advocates, too, have urged its inclusion into the oral curriculum. Lowell (personal communication, January 1981), the Director of the John Tracy Clinic in Los Angeles, though more cautious, sees great merit in investigating the effectiveness of the written language approach in the oral curriculum.

Aside from teaching written language directly to young children, there has also been little research in teaching reading and written language to young preschool-age hearing-impaired children, even where the medium of speech or sign language is used. I am aware of only two studies that employ sign language (Williams, 1968, in teaching the reading of English, and Söderbergh, 1976, in teaching the reading of Swedish) and of only one that uses speech as the means of instruction (Lado, 1972, in teaching the reading of English). The fact that so little research has been devoted to such an important problem is perhaps the result of attitudes prevailing in society at large concerning whether children should be taught to read at an early age. Hearing children, particularly in America, are not thought to have sufficiently developed intellectual capacities. A number of studies do show, however, that given proper instruction, hearing children can acquire substantial reading knowledge and skills, even those as young as 1 and 2 years of age. The long-term studies of Söderbergh (1971), Weeks (in press), Doman (1964), Durkin (1970, 1974), Steinberg (1980), and Steinberg and Steinberg (1975), for example, provide support for this view. Such research further demonstrates that current reading readiness tests for English are quite invalid and underestimate the age at which children are ready to read. Essentially, the sort of knowledge and skills that are demanded of children in these tests are mainly irrelevant to the learning of reading. (See Steinberg, 1980, for a detailed examination of the readiness issue.)

In light of the considerations discussed

above, there is strong reason to believe that hearing-impaired children, provided they do not have serious cognitive disabilities, will benefit from being taught written language and reading in their early years. What is necessary is an appropriate conceptual foundation and methodology that is suitable to their needs.

THEORETICAL GUIDING PRINCIPLES

For the learning and teaching of written language by the hearing impaired, four basic theoretical principles may serve as guides: (a) A nonsound environment can provide a sufficient conceptual foundation for the learning of written language, (b) the understanding of written language provides the necessary foundation for the expression of written language, (c) words are best acquired as conceptual wholes in a relevant context, and (d) phrases and sentences are best acquired in a relevant context through induction.

The nonsound environment

Before considering the situation of the hearing impaired, it may be instructive to first consider the situation of hearing persons acquiring language. Initially, speech sounds convey no ideas to young hearing children, but after a period of time, they do. Consideration of this phenomenon clearly indicates that hearing only speech sounds is insufficient for the acquisition of meaning. What the learner requires is some environmental experience besides the speech sounds themselves to provide clues to meaning. No matter how many times children heard the word *dog*, for example, they would not know that such sounds signal the object or idea of a dog. It is essential that some object, situation, or event be experienced in conjunction with the speech sounds for meaning to be acquired. Of course, once a certain amount of language has been learned, this previously learned language itself may be used to explain the meaning of new words. However, the ultimate source of the meanings of the words used in such explanations, it should be recognized, involves some nonspeech experience that is essential to the formation of concepts. The extensive research of Piaget and his associates, it might be noted, provides support for this view of language acquisition (Piaget, 1955; Piaget & Inhelder, 1969; Sinclair, 1970). Actually, even the innate ideas view of Chomsky (MacIntyre, 1970) is not in disagreement with this conception, since his theory also requires that certain relevant environmental events occur before innate ideas become activated and functional. Children still need to experience objects such as dogs and cats to be able to understand the speech sounds used to represent those objects.

To the extent that hearing-impaired children experience the same nonsound environment as hearing children, they can acquire the same concepts relating to that

---

Only concepts and experiences that relate to sound will be denied to the hearing impaired, much the same as color and visual shapes are denied to the blind.

environment. Their experiences can then be associated with written forms, so that in time such forms acquire a symbolic value, that is, meaning. Only concepts and experiences that relate to sound, such as music, noise, and sounds of nature, will be denied to the hearing impaired, much the same as color and visual shapes are denied to the blind.

Written language understanding

Again, one must first consider the situation for hearing persons. In acquiring language, hearing persons learn to understand speech before they produce it meaningfully. Not surprisingly, children do not utter words or sentences meaningfully until they first hear and understand the words and sentences that others have spoken (Huttenlocher, 1974; Sachs & Truswell, 1976; de Villiers & de Villiers, 1978). Of course, they often imitate words, as do parrots, but this in itself is not regarded as meaningful language use or understanding.

As far as the hearing-impaired child who is learning written language is concerned, a similar primacy of understanding over production can be expected. In this case, however, understanding would consist of the interpretation of written forms, and production would consist of the writing of forms. Thus, a child would have to learn to interpret (understand) written forms before being able to produce them in any meaningful way. Production would, therefore, lag behind understanding. It might be noted that an even greater lag in writing production may be expected compared with the lag that occurs in speech. The muscle and coordination controls needed for the use of a writing implement develop much slower than the articulators used in the production of speech. Children typically only begin to gain control of a writing implement around the age of 3 years (Steinberg & Yamada, 1980), and it takes some years before they can write numbers of sentences without tiring. This is unfortunate, for hearing-impaired children could benefit greatly through using such a communicative means of expression during their early years.

Word acquisition

Once a hearing-impaired child begins to acquire concepts of objects, actions, events, and situations, that child is ready to acquire the written labels for these concepts. Undoubtedly, the ideal way for a young hearing-impaired child to learn words in their written form is in much the same way as the young hearing child does: exposure to words in conjunction with the objects, situations, and ongoing events in the environment. Unfortunately, it is easy for a parent to produce spoken words while conducting the affairs of daily life, but it is difficult for written words to be produced in that situation. The practical obstacles for a parent to write everything that he or she would ordinarily say are so formidable that even a limited attempt has little chance of success.

Since conditions for learning cannot be arranged so that hearing-impaired children can learn written language on their own in the ordinary course of daily events as do hearing children, some form of explicit teaching must be provided. However, although some degree of artificiality must be introduced into the acquisition situation, the simulation of naturalness should be a goal. Language learning should be made to occur indirectly through the course of interesting activities and games and not through explicit language lessons. The teaching of vocabulary and syntax are considered from this perspective.

When teaching how to write words, it is proposed that the best approach is to teach words as wholes and not as parts and that the words that are taught are ones for which the child already has the concept. Two reasons are offered for this position: the inappropriateness of an analytic approach (particularly for young children) and the greater ease of learning of meaningful units.

Inappropriateness of an analytic approach

When hearing children experience speech words in the home, they experience them as wholes; the words *dog* and *cat*, for example, are pronounced as wholes. The child is not taught the component sounds first, for example, /d/, /a/, and /g/. Rather, parents say whole words like *dogs*, *jumped*, and *runs* and leave it to the children to make the syllable and morpheme segmentation on their own. The children accomplish this through a natural analytical process of their own—induction. Since evidence shows that the analytical and conceptualizing processes of hearing-impaired children do not differ from those of hearing children (Furth, 1971), hearing-impaired children may be expected to be able to distinguish on their own the shapes of the letters and to identify morpheme components of words in the course of learning whole written words. There is no need, therefore, to give prior (or even subsequent) training on individual letters and sounds to hearing-impaired children, training that is exceedingly tedious and difficult for children. Such training is inappropriate for written language education. All that the child need be exposed to is a written word and a meaning.

Greater ease of learning meaningful written units

Although a word is longer and more complex than any of its component parts, research evidence indicates that the learning of a meaningful whole word is easier than the learning of its meaningless components. In an experiment with American preschool children, Steinberg and Kono (1979) found that words were learned at more than twice the rate of letters. Similar findings have been found for Japanese children, who learned complex Chinese characters at least twice as quickly as meaningless syllable symbols (Steinberg & Yamada, 1978–1979). Thus, children will learn written items if those items are associated with meaningful stimuli; meaningful stimuli, such as actual objects, events, and situations (or their pictures), can be paired with the written items for hearing-impaired children. Thus, if a written word is associated with a cookie or a picture of a dog, the hearing-impaired child can be expected to acquire the written forms that represent those objects. To the extent that the associated stimulus is not meaningful, the written item is much more difficult to learn.

Insofar as the learning of abstract words

is concerned, no special principles need be followed. The hearing-impaired child will learn to acquire such words in essentially the same way as does the hearing child, that is, on the basis of relevant environmental experience and through a process of hypothesis testing. Abstract words like *cause*, *idea*, *like*, *beautiful*, *pain*, *true*, and *wish* begin to be acquired after children come to realize the essential principle of language, which is that words can be used to express ideas. This basic principle is acquired through the learning of concrete words. After this, the child is ready to label more abstract notions.

Phrase and sentence acquisition

Just as hearing children learn the syntax of language without direct instruction by exposure to phrases and sentences used in a relevant environmental context, hearing-impaired children learn the syntax of written language in the same way. Parents of hearing children do not teach their children syntactic rules. For example, rules about constituent order, verb inflections, and relative clause formation are learned by children on their own. Explanations would not be understood by the young child, even if the simplest language were used. Imagine, for example, trying to explain the use of *to* and *at* to a 3- or 4-year-old. The child would not be able to understand the explanation, even if the parent could give it correctly! Only advanced speakers of a language with mature abstract intellectual capacity can benefit by grammatical explanations. Such being the case, parents and instructors should attempt to provide the hearing-impaired child with adequate exposure to written language and environmental stimuli in as natural and interesting a way as possible. Through such exposure, the children can then be expected to learn the syntax by themselves through induction and hypothesis testing.

A PROGRAM FOR TEACHING WRITTEN LANGUAGE

A four-phase teaching program was formulated incorporating the principles previously outlined. The four phases were (a) word familiarization, (b) word identification, (c) phrase and sentence identification, and (d) text interpretation, with all but the last phase being applied to the subject before termination of the project.

General instructions

Four teaching instructions are common to all phases. First, whenever possible, the instructor should point to the written words in a left to right fashion (underneath or to the side of the word so as not to block its view). The children are to be encouraged to point in a similar manner. In this way, children will get used to the idea that words are to be perceived in a certain direction. Second, children should never be required to say what is written. Only if they are able and willing should they do so. Otherwise, demanding a speech response will greatly slow the acquisition process. On the other hand, although it is not directly part of this program, the instructor is advised to pronounce (or sign, if that medium is available) what is written. In this way the children may benefit from other forms of language input (to the extent that such forms are perceived). Third, children should not be required to write as part of the program. The fine motor coordination that is needed to write letters is difficult for a young child. If such a skill were made a part of the comprehension procedure, then the rate at which a child could learn to understand words will be retarded. This is not to say that learning to write is not an essential ability for the child to acquire. It most certainly is. The point is that the teaching of writing should not be included in procedures that aim to teach the understanding of written items. The teaching of writing may be done, but at another time. Fourth, children should enjoy written language activities; what is boring and tedious should be avoided.

Phase 1: word familiarization

The purpose of this phase is to acquaint children with the forms of written words and to make them aware that different written words relate to different objects. Children are not required to remember, however, which particular written word is associated with which particular object. Such learning is reserved for the next phase, word identification.

First, words are written on blank cards by the instructor and are attached to familiar objects or pictures in all of the rooms that the child frequents. The cards are placed at the child's eye level wherever possible. The instructor points to the object (e.g., a chair) and then points to the written word. In this way, the children come to realize that different written words are associated with different objects. Just seeing the cards repeatedly will enable the children to identify written words on their own without explicit teaching. In conjunction with the word cards around the room, a variety of games may be played.

Word familiarization games and activities should be continued until the child can identify a written word without the presence of any clue. This feat is called identification. The length of time required will generally depend on the age of the child. Individual differences are to be expected, just as they are with hearing children in language learning.

Phase 2: word identification

In this phase, the children learn which particular written words are associated with which particular objects. The difference between this phase and the preceding one is that this requires the use of long-term memory. Here the children must store a particular written configuration and remember what particular object it represents. No clues are given as is done in the familiarization phase.

Since there is virtually no end to acquiring vocabulary, this phase is continued even after phrases and sentences are introduced. Phrases and sentences may be introduced when children have acquired a sufficient number of nouns, verbs, adjectives, or adverbs (e.g., *car* and *red*) so that phrases or sentences can be formed with them (e.g., "red car" and "Give me the red car").

Phase 3: phrase and sentence identification

This phase is similar to word identification except that larger linguistic units are introduced. The goal is for children to

It is best not to create phrases and sentences for their own sake but to make them fit the events and situations that occur in the immediate environment.

---

read the basic linguistic unit that expresses propositions, that is, the sentence, of which words and phrases are components. Learning such units promotes the apprehension of meaning, which word-by-word reading tends to reduce. As much as possible, phrases and sentences are to be composed of the single words that have already been learned, since too many unknown words may cause frustration and make learning difficult.

Phrases such as "red car" and sentences such as "Alice fell" could be introduced as soon as some of the main component words are learned. It is best not to create phrases and sentences for their own sake, however, but to make them fit the events and situations that occur in the immediate environment. The sentence *Alice fell* would be of great interest to a child if the child did observe Alice fall.

Phase 4: text interpretation

Text is the largest meaningful written linguistic unit, consisting of a sequence of two or more sentences that are semantically and syntactically related to one another. (The prior phase dealt only with sentences in isolation.) Learning to interpret text may be the most interesting of all activities for children, since there is an excitement that a story can generate but that isolated words, phrases, and sentences cannot. It is the purpose of this phase to provide children with the knowledge and skill that will enable them to interpret text fluently.

Just when text teaching should be introduced on a serious basis is difficult to say. Some knowledge of words, phrases, and sentences is certainly required so that proceeding through a book is made easy, but what this amount should be is a matter of conjecture. As an estimate, 50 words and 20 phrases and sentences might suffice, depending on the simplicity of the items in the book. In addition, children should have reached the stage at which they are beginning to understand new sentences that involve a substitution of members in a word class. Thus, given that a child has learned the meaning of *boy* and of *The girl jumped*, the child should be able to comprehend *The boy jumped* without ever having seen this sentence before. Until such a level of knowledge is attained, text interpretation might be too difficult a task.

Activities involving text other than that in books may also be introduced. For example, stories with as few as two or three sentences may be composed (e.g., Story 1: (a) Alice dropped the egg; (b) It landed on the dog. Story 2: (a) Mike was riding a bicycle; (b) He hit a rock; (c) The bicycle turned over). Each sentence of a story may be written on a card, along with a corresponding picture. One activity could be for children to arrive at the order of sentences that form the story. The pictures on the cards could later be removed as the children learn to understand the meaning of the sentences.

Books for children can be custom-made or store bought. Each has its advantages.

The custom-made book can be composed directly of vocabulary that a child knows. Then, too, the child can help in its making. On the other hand, although the store-bought book may not have a completely appropriate vocabulary or syntax, such books are attractive and may well stimulate and broaden a child's interest.

As children progress linguistically and intellectually, so too should such advancement be reflected in the books they are given. Selections should be carefully made for them until the time when they are able to make suitable selections on their own. It should be noted that although this phase is concerned with the teaching of text from books, it is not recommended that the introduction of books be delayed until this phase is reached. Children can enjoy and learn much about books long before the serious teaching of their linguistic content is begun.

EFFECTIVENESS OF THE TEACHING PROGRAM

To date, I have been involved in teaching written language to four children on the basis of the four-phase teaching program. Two are boys, Jerrold and Konrad, and two are girls, Jessie and Kiku. At the program's inception, the ages of the children were: Jerrold, 3 years 6 months; Konrad, 2 years 5 months; Jessie, 1 year 2 months; and Kiku, 1 year 5 months. The first three children are Americans who are learning English in Hawaii; the fourth, Kiku, is a Japanese learning Japanese in Japan. In all cases, teaching was done by family members in the home. All items taught were selected by them.

All of the children are profoundly deaf, having a 90-dB or higher hearing loss in their better ear. Except for one American child, Jerrold, who became deaf due to meningitis at age 5 months, the children have had no significant hearing since birth. The main criterion for subject selection was their profound hearing loss. It was believed that a great loss would give the program its most rigorous test, since such children would be likely to acquire only a small amount of language through residual hearing. Not surprisingly, therefore, at the beginning of the study, the linguistic knowledge of the children was at a minimum. Only the two boys had any linguistic knowledge at all. Jerrold, the oldest, could say about 15 words and understood about 40 spoken words. He also could understand about 15 word signs. The other, Konrad, knew no speech but could understand about 8 words in sign language. Some of the more important characteristics of the subjects and their families are shown in Table 1, as are the overall results.

Thus, it can be seen that Konrad learned the greatest number of items (648) and Jessie the least (5). Undoubtedly, factors such as the length of the instruction period and the average amount of time spent daily on instruction (parents' reported estimates) played a role in determining the number of items learned. For example, it seems that Jerrold might have learned many more items than he did had he received as much daily instruction and for as long a period of time as did Konrad. Incidentally, instruction was never given in a single block of time; it was spaced throughout the day. Whether age is also a factor affecting the rate of learning cannot be determined from the data in the chart

Table 1. Background of American and Japanese subjects and number of items learned

Variable	Jerrold	Konrad	Jessie	Kiku
Written language learned	English	English	English	Japanese
Sex	Male	Male	Female	Female
Age at program beginning	3 yr., 6 mo.	2 yr., 5 mo.	1 yr., 2 mo.	1 yr., 5 mo.
Hearing loss in better ear	Over 90 dB	Over 90 dB	Around 90 dB	Around 90 dB
Hearing loss onset	5 months	Congenital	Congenital	Congenital
Etiology	Meningitis	Unknown	Unknown	Unknown
Father's occupation	Engineer	Sewage worker	Mechanic	Engineer
Mother's occupation	Computer programmer	Homemaker	Office head	Homemaker
Father's education	University	Jr. high school	University	University
Mother's education	University	Jr. high school	University	University
Duration of instruction	11 mo.	15 mo.	8 mo.	20 mo.
Average daily instruction	10 min.	30 min.	30 min.	25 min.
Single words learned	180	406	5	194
Phrases, expressions, sentences learned	134	242	—	96
Total items learned	314	648	5	290

alone, since achievement could be due to other sources. For example, differences in teaching effectiveness on the part of the parents as well as differences in the age of innate intellectual ability of the children could have contributed to the observed results.

• • •

The results show that significant written language knowledge, even of such vastly different writing systems as English and Japanese, can be acquired directly through the medium of writing by very young children who have had a profound hearing loss at or near birth. Since the written language teaching program can be applied successfully by ordinary parents in the home, there is good reason to believe that it can also be successfully applied by teachers in school. Undoubtedly, young children would benefit most by being taught written language in both the home and the school. However, it seems more appropriate that the program should have its foundation in the school. Not all parents can easily learn what is necessary to help their children, nor may they be sufficiently motivated. Then, too, practical considerations may prevent adequate parent participation, such as when both parents work. For those parents who can teach in the home, training and direction can best be provided by a school staff. Such a day may not be far off if programs to teach written language are incorporated into the curricula of schools for the hearing impaired.

REFERENCES

Bell, A.G. Upon a method of teaching language to a very young congenitally deaf child. *American Annals of the Deaf and Dumb,* 1883, *28*(3), 124–139.

Dalgarno, G. *Didascalocophus, or the deaf and dumb man's tutor.* Menston, England: Scolar Press, 1971. (Originally published by Theatre in Oxford, Oxford, England, 1680.)

de Villiers, J.G., & de Villiers, P.A. *Language acquisition.* Cambridge, Mass.: Harvard University Press, 1978.

Doman, G. *How to teach your baby to read.* New York: Random House, 1964.

Durkin, D. A language arts program for pre-first grade children: Two-year achievement report. *Reading Research Quarterly,* 1970, *5,* 534–565.

Durkin, D. A six-year study of children who learned to read in school at the age of four. *Reading Research Quarterly,* 1974, *10,* 9–61.

Furth, H.G. *Thinking without language.* New York: Free Press, 1966.

Furth, H.G. Linguistic deficiency and thinking: Research with deaf subjects, 1964–1969. *Psychological Bulletin,* 1971, *76,* 58–72.

Huttenlocher, J. The origins of language comprehension. In R.L. Solso (Ed.), *Theories in cognitive psychology.* Potomac, Md.: Erlbaum, 1974.

Lado, R. Early reading by a child with severe hearing loss as an aid to linguistic and intellectual development. *Georgetown University Papers on Languages and Linguistics,* 1972, *6,* 1–6.

Lado, R. Early reading as language development. *Georgetown University Papers on Languages and Linguistics,* 1976, *13,* 8–15.

Lane, H.S., & Baker, D. Reading achievement of the deaf: Another look. *Volta Review,* November 1974, *76,* 489–499.

Lenneberg, E. Prerequisites for language acquisition by the deaf. In T.J. O'Rourke (Ed.), Psycholinguistics and total communication: The state of the art. *American Annals of the Deaf,* 1972. (Monograph).

MacIntyre, A. Noam Chomsky's view of language. In M. Lester (Ed.), *Readings in applied transformational grammar* (2nd ed.). New York: Holt, Rinehart & Winston, 1970.

Piaget, J. *The language and thought of the child.* Cleveland, Ohio: World, 1955.

Piaget, J. & Inhelder, B. *The psychology of the child.* New York: Basic Books, 1969.

Sachs, J.S., & Truswell, L. Comprehension of two-word instructions by children in the one-word stage. *Papers and Reports on Child Language,* 1976, *12,* 212–220.

Sinclair, H. The transition from sensory-motor behavior to symbolic activity. *Interchange,* 1970, *1,* 119–126.

Söderbergh, R. *Reading in early childhood.* Stockholm, Sweden: Almquist & Wiksell, 1971. (Reprinted by Georgetown University Press, Washington, D.C., 1977.)

Söderbergh, R. Learning to read between two and five: Some observations on normal hearing and deaf children. *Stockholm Universitet Monograph: Institutionen for Nordiska Spraak,* 1976 (Preprint No. 12).

Steinberg, D.D. *Teaching reading to nursery school. Final report.* (Grant No. G007903113). Washington, D.C.: Office of Education, U.S. Department of Education, 1980.

Steinberg, D.D., & Kono, R. *Working Papers in Linguistics* (University of Hawaii), 1979, *9,* 3, 115–117.

Steinberg, D.D., & Steinberg, M.T. Reading before speaking. *Visible Language,* 1975, *9,* 197–224.

Steinberg, D.D., & Yamada, J. Are whole word *kanji* easier to learn than syllable *kana? Reading Research Quarterly,* 1978–79, *14,* 1, 88–99.

Steinberg, D.D., & Yamada, J. [The ability of young children to write.] *Kyooiku Sinrigaku Kenkyuu,* 1980, *28,* 4.

Weeks, T. Early childhood literacy. *Encounters with language.* Rowley, Mass.: Newbury House, in press.

Williams, J.S. Bilingual experiences of a deaf child. (ERIC Document Reproduction Service No. ED 030 092) 1968.

Wrightstone, J.W., Aronow, M.S., & Moskowitz, S. Developing reading test norms for deaf children. *American Annals of the Deaf,* 1963, *108,* 311–316.

Amplification: tool for language skills

Mark Ross, PhD
Professor
Department of Communication Sciences
University of Connecticut
Storrs, Connecticut

APPROPRIATELY delivered amplified sound is the most effective therapy tool available for most hearing-impaired children. This is an assertion that relatively few professionals may accept as stated; most would agree that proper amplification is a valuable tool but perhaps not the most effective one. For these individuals, the application of amplification in therapy takes place alongside, and equal to, other intervention strategies, such as speech and language therapy, academic tutoring, classroom management, and parent counseling. All of these are vital, particularly, the parent component in a parent–infant program. In spite of their undoubted value, none address in a direct fashion the reason for concern with the child in the first place. Only amplification addresses the problem at its source, which is the hearing loss. Applied early and appropriately, with due consideration for the many factors that can minimize its import, amplification will produce more progress in the dimensions in which the child is handicapped (speech, language, academic, and possibly in the psychosocial areas as well) than any of these other therapies. The assertion, therefore, is not being made as a deliberately extremist position, with the intention that a fall-back position would still result in a more auditorially oriented therapy practice than is now generally the case. It is the therapy of choice for most hearing-impaired children simply because it can pay the most dividends.

AUDITORY CHANNEL

The auditory channel on which normal communication is ordinarily based is the normal route through which speech and language develop. The biological propensity of human beings to evolve a communication system through audition is well documented (Fry, 1978). Hearing-impaired children possess the same biological potential to develop speech and language as do normal hearing children. What they lack is a sufficient quantity and quality of amplified linguistic input in the appropriate nonlinguistic circumstances. The argument that hearing-impaired children, by virtue of their hearing losses, must depend on alternative means of developing a communication system, and thus forego the usual route, is true for only a small percentage of the general population of hearing-impaired children. The overwhelming majority possess some residual hearing (Office of Demographic Studies, 1971); most of this latter group have sufficient residual hearing so that when used effectively, the auditory channel can still serve as the primary channel for communication purposes. Any child with any residual hearing can derive some benefit from amplified sound even though for those with the most profound losses, audition may only serve as a supplement to a primarily visual mode of communication. There are within the general population of hearing-impaired children, 15 to 20 times more who can be classified as hard of hearing, those for whom the auditory channel can serve as the primary mode for communication purposes as there are "deaf" children (i.e., those for whom the auditory channel can be quite important, but *not* primary) (Ross & Giolas, 1978).

The first step, then, in realizing the contribution of residual hearing for all hearing-impaired children is to acknowledge what it can and cannot do and agree that whatever benefit it can offer in interpersonal communication has merit. The second step relates to the factors that can either diminish or enhance the utilization of residual hearing. These include sensory deprivation effects, maintenance of hearing aids, electroacoustic adjustments, binaural hearing, classroom acoustics, and the use of auditory trainers. The third step is subsumed under the title "auditory training," though not in a traditional sense.

AUDITORY SENSORY DEPRIVATION

One of the most crucial variables in building the auditory potential is time. If amplification is delayed, if no speech signals enter into and stimulate the auditory system while the child is still young, then

> *One of the most crucial variables in building the auditory potential is time.*

that system will exhibit physiological and morphological changes that will limit its function and at some point in time become irreversible. The evidence for this statement is derived mainly by analogy from animal research and some inferences from the behavior of children with early conductive losses (Clopton & Silverman, 1977; Patchett, 1977; Webster & Webster, 1977.)

How long such deprivation must last with children before the effect occurs or is reversible is not known. It is probable that it occurs on a time continuum; the longer the deprivation, the greater the effects. Some restoration of function is possible even with prolonged delay in human beings, as long as the central nervous system still retains a good deal of neural plasticity. I have seen children who apparently made effective use of amplified sound when their first experience was at age 9 or 10 years. I have fitted aids on some motivated "deaf" adults who found the experience of sound helpful in controlling their own speech output and in assisting their speech reading. In both of these instances, however, it is likely that amplified speech sounds would have provided more information had the amplification begun much earlier (by 6 or 8 months of age).

A recent body of literature evaluating the effects of chronic otitis media in children has developed (Gottlieb, Zinkus, & Thompson, 1979; Kessler & Randolph, 1979; Masters & Marsh, 1978; Zinkus & Gottlieb, 1980). The general consensus of these studies is that such children demonstrate significant deficiencies in auditory sequential memory, phonemic synthesis, reading, phonology, and some language skills. They also receive much more remedial help in schools than children without an early history of middle ear problems. Many children with middle ear problems experience intermittent periods of deprivation; hearing becomes an unstable avenue for building a basic perceptual framework. The dimensions that are purely auditory suffer more than those visually mediated. Behavior that has been labeled a *learning disorder* occurs more frequently with them.

The animal and human literature strongly suggests that much of the failures or reduced significance of using amplified sound can be directly attributed to delays in providing such sound exposure. This does not only affect children with severe or profound losses or those with early fluctuating hearing loss, but also those children with moderate or severe high-frequency losses. For these children, sound may be experienced at some low frequencies at any early age, but stimulation of the important high frequencies may not occur until appropriately adjusted amplification is achieved. This may not happen (if ever) until the child is in elementary school. In other words, sensory deprivation may affect certain frequencies but not others because sound sensations do not occur naturally. The tonotopic organization of the auditory system, in which certain areas of the cochlea, eighth nerve, and midbrain auditory nuclei are responsive primarily to certain frequencies and not others, lends support to the assumption that sensory deprivation effects can be frequency specific. Limiting the function of these high frequencies, which carry much of the consonantal energy in speech, has grave implications for speech perception and, thus, language develpment. Speech sound energy, then, not only has to be experienced early but also has to be delivered to much of the residual hearing range of the individual up to at least 6000 KHz.

HEARING AID MAINTENANCE

Since the first systematic investigation of children's hearing aids in schools over 15 years ago (Gaeth & Lounsbury, 1966), the topic has been evaluated on a number of occasions by other investigators (see Ross, 1977, for a review). The consensus of these results is that approximately 30% to 40% of the aids checked could be considered to be functioning poorly, if at all. Most of the problems were easy to detect, including such malfunctions as weak or dead batteries, the aid turned on the "off" or "T" position, excessive distortion, and no sound amplification at all. Earmold-related problems were also apparent, such as blockage of the sound channel by cerumen, improper seating of the mold in the ear, and the occurrence of acoustic feedback. All of these malfunctions are easy to detect, and most can be corrected easily. They will not be, however, unless a daily, systematic troubleshooting program is instituted.

The point to remember about children's hearing aids is that almost anything can go wrong and usually will. The eventual goal is to make the children themselves responsible for the operation of the hearing aid. But unless the process is taken seriously and shown to be important, they are not likely to. A daily troubleshooting program can be effective and can markedly reduce the occurrence of malfunctions, as several recent studies have shown (Bendet, 1980; Kenker, McConnell, Logan, & Green, 1979). The equipment necessary is minimal—just a battery tester, a hearing aid stethoscope, and the examiner's ears. It is helpful initially to have a checklist of possible problems available and to keep longitudinal records of the adequacy of each child's hearing aid. Detailed troubleshooting procedures and checklists can be found in Ross, Brackett, and Maxon (1982).

ELECTROACOUSTIC ADJUSTMENTS

Wearing a hearing aid that is operating does not mean that it is properly adjusted. Unfortunately, relatively little attention is paid to ensure that the pattern of amplified sound received by children conveys the maximum acoustic information that they are capable of receiving. This is not a trivial matter. One would hardly accept a few standard refractions in eyeglasses, and one should not accept its auditory analogy. The children seen in schools and clinics exhibit a range of losses differing in degree and slope, among other dimensions, and the sound amplification requirement decisions must take their individual needs into consideration. A hearing aid may be operating perfectly but still not be appropriate for a particular child.

First example

Consider Figure 1. The unaided sound-field thresholds for the right ear are shown by the circles. It is obvious that the residual hearing of this child, a boy, is concentrated in the low frequencies. He is a profoundly deaf child, of a type whose capacity to profit from amplified sound is generally underestimated. Now consider the dimension indicated by triangles. This is the output of his hearing aid to a 70-dB sound-field speech spectrum input. To make the example clearer, both of these dimensions have been plotted on the same reference level. It can be noted that the

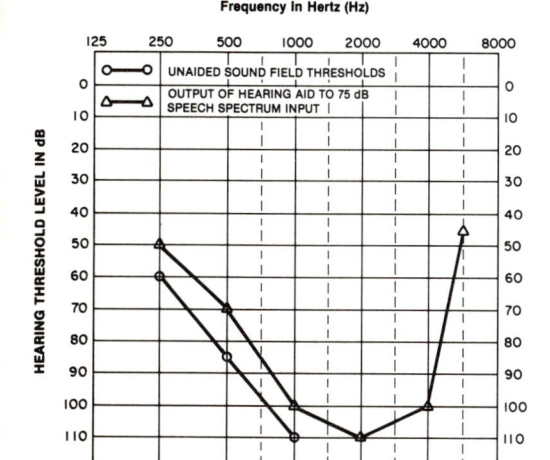

Figure 1. Unaided sound-field audiogram and output of a hearing aid plotted on the same reference level. (The triangles indicate the sound pressure output delivered by the hearing aid to a 75-dB speech spectrum input; the circles indicate the threshold of hearing.)

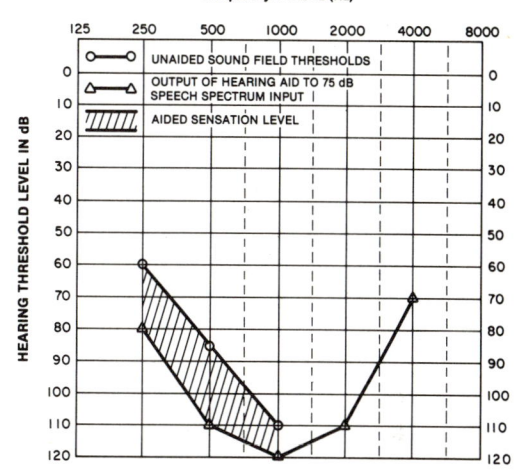

Figure 2. Output of a hearing aid plotted in reference to the unaided sound-field thresholds. (The cross-hatched area indicates the sensation level across frequency resulting from the amplified speech signal.)

output of the aid does not reach the threshold of the child. Nevertheless, it is a perfectly functioning hearing aid. When listened to by a teacher or parent with normal hearing, it appears to provide adequate sound amplification. The child's lack of or only occasional responses to sound than supports the preconceived notion that sound amplification in a child like this is hardly worth bothering with. With the hearing aid appearing to be virtually useless, the real training of the child proceeds to focus on visual inputs. However, now consider the same child with a different hearing aid, adjusted to provide a more suitable amplified signal to the same sound-field speech spectrum input (see Figure 2).

The line connected by triangles again indicates the output of the hearing aid. It can be noted that it now exceeds the child's thresholds at 250, 500, and 1000 Hz by 20, 25, and 10 dB, respectively. Sound is being detected consistently by the child, but only at the low frequencies. Still these sensations can be of great value in the perception and production of speech, particularly if the child is exposed to them at an early age, before sensory deprivation limits the potential auditory contribution.

With this much residual hearing, this child should be able to hear the first formant of all of the vowels and the second formants of some of the back and midvowels. The low-frequency nasality cue is available to him. He should be able to differentiate voice from voiceless consonants on the basis of their characteristic voice onset times before and after vowels. He may be able to perceive the presence of some of the plosive consonants as they modify the second-formant transitions of the midvowels and back vowels, even though the consonant energy itself is not audible. The semivowels and liquids, with their characteristically long and slow formant transitions, can be differentiated auditorily from other phonemes. The prosody of speech, incorporating changes in stress, intonation, duration, and rhythmical groupings of speech, is conveyed by the low frequencies. This suprasegmental information can also aid in decoding the meaning of certain utterances, such as questions versus statements and *per*mit versus per*mit*, and it assists in separating grammatical groupings in the flow of speech (Levitt, 1978; Ling, 1978a; Pickett, 1980). The speech reading process can be significantly fostered with the availability of this much acoustic information, with auditory self-monitoring helping the development of more intelligible speech.

Second example

A child with much more residual hearing is portrayed in Figures 3–5. In Figure 3, the circles again indicate the unaided sound-field thresholds, and the triangles again show the output of the hearing aid to a 70-dB sound-field speech spectrum input. As can be noted, the resulting pattern of amplified sensation levels (the level of the sound delivered above the unaided sound-field thresholds) is concentrated in the low frequencies. This is not a desirable pattern of amplification. As a matter of fact, this child is receiving essentially the same sensation levels at the same frequencies as the child in the previous example. Yet she has much more potentially usable and valuable residual hearing. Certainly, the amplification system that she is wearing will permit her to hear, but she will

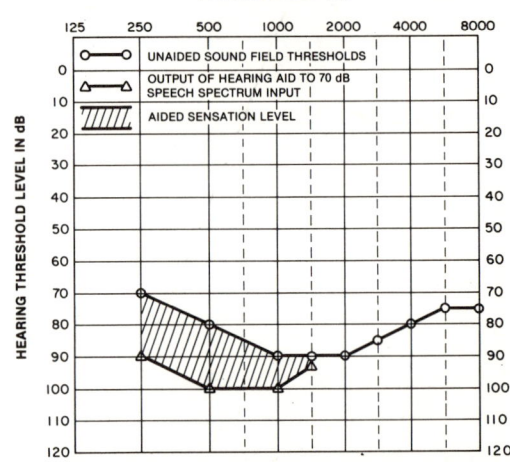

Figure 3. More potential residual hearing than in Figures 1 and 2. (However, output of the hearing aid to a 75-dB speech spectrum input is concentrated in the low frequencies. Actual amplified residual hearing is similar to the previous example.)

also undoubtedly demonstrate severe speech and language deficits. Furthermore, what frequently occurs in cases like this is that emphasis is placed directly on the observable behavior, with too little awareness of the underlying cause—a poor amplification system.

Figure 4 is an example of a different pattern of amplification with the same child. In this example, the maximum output of the hearing aid is set too low. At maximum, the resulting sensation levels are barely 5–10 dB across frequencies. This does not present sufficient acoustical raw material for optimal speech and language development through the auditory channel. (Sometimes due to concern that overamplification may produce permanent threshold shifts, the opposite extreme is reached wherein sufficient amplification is not provided. At any rate, the evidence regarding the effect of hearing aid amplification on residual hearing does not give cause for alarm regarding this effect, though caution should always be exercised. (See Ross & Giolas, 1978, pp. 256–259, for a review of the topic.) In this example, the remedial measure is obvious: Increase the output of the electroacoustic system.

Figure 5 presents an optimal amplification pattern across frequency for the same subject. There is somewhat less of an amplified sensation level at the lower frequencies than the higher frequencies, since these lower frequencies may render the higher frequencies less audible (Danaher & Pickett, 1975). At the same time, the frequency range is extended to 6000 Hz, ensuring the audibility of the important high-frequency information in speech, such as the /s/ phoneme.

Each of the above three examples illustrates different patterns of amplified sound for the same child. It cannot be expected that each of these systems would be equally useful. The concept of amplifi-

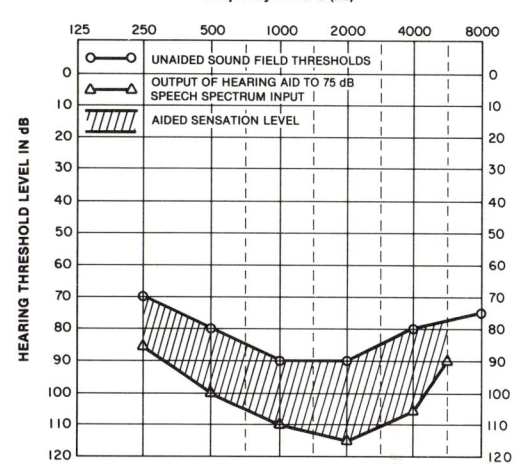

Figure 5. Output of the hearing aid to a speech spectrum input (now provides adequate amplification across frequency up to 6000 Hz).

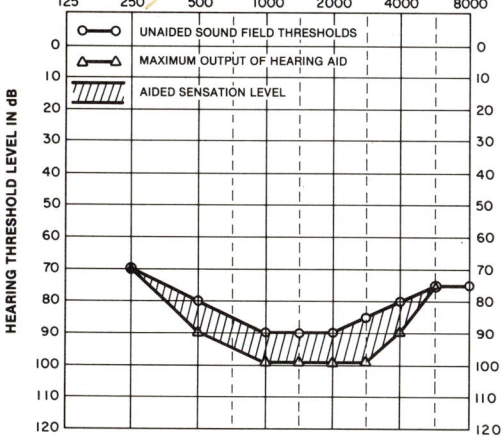

Figure 4. Output of the hearing aid (provides only a 5- to 10-dB sensation level across frequency).

> *After many years of research with hearing aids and literally thousands of publications, the conclusion seems to be that the more sound available to the person, the better that person hears.*

cation as a tool for linguistic growth must begin with increasing the audibility of the speech signal across the widest possible frequency range. There are qualifications and exceptions to this (see Ross et al., 1982, for a complete discussion), but the general rule does hold. The profession of audiology is beginning to recognize that the most important determiner of intelligibility when wearing hearing aids is the extent and breadth with which the amplified signal exceeds either a noise floor or the person's acuity thresholds (Dugal, Braida, & Durlach, 1980; Studebaker & Wark, 1980). After many years of research with hearing aids and literally thousands of publications, the conclusion seems to be that the more sound available to the person, the better that person hears.

There are many different ways of obtaining a desired amplification pattern, the most common being making tonal adjustments in the hearing aid/auditory trainer. Recently, there has been a great deal of emphasis in making these adjustments and achieving a desired amplified sensation level through the use of acoustic dampers in the tone hooks and modifications in the bore diameters of the tubing and earmold. The acoustic dampers act to smooth out the real-ear (measured in the canal with a probe microphone or with aided sound-field testing) response by reducing response irregularities, and the bore diameter modifications act to increase the effective frequency range of the entire electroacoustic system (Killion, 1981). Most hearing aid users of postauricular hearing aids should be able to increase their detection of speech sounds to some extent with these new types of earmolds (Libby, Johnson, & Longwell, 1981).

BINAURAL HEARING AIDS

Binaural hearing aids involve electroacoustic adjustments to both ears simultaneously rather than to each ear separately. In some circles, the concept of providing children with a hearing aid for each ear is still questionable. This is an unfortunate attitude, which leads to children making less effective use of their residual hearing than is possible (see Ross, 1980; Ross & Giolas, 1978, pp. 261–268).

The research on this topic can be summarized by saying that generally speaking, a binaural fitting will provide more auditory information to the person than a single aid. (See Libby, 1980, for an extensive review.) Most hearing-impaired people who wear two aids show improved speech discrimination skills, localization ability, and binaural summation of loudness compared to those using only one aid. Subjectively, they experience enhanced loudness, they work less hard to achieve speech comprehension, and one ear is always in a relatively favorable position to detect speech signals. In cases in which there is assymetrical but usable hearing in each ear, the brain is supplied with different auditory information from both ears to enhance the total perception of sound. This same concept is employed in cases of bilateral symmetrical losses in which the frequency responses of the two hearing aids are differentially modified. In terms of the signal-to-noise concept, binaural aids permit someone to function as if there were approximately 3 dB more signal present than would be the case if only a monaural aid were used, which can make a significant difference in the comprehension of speech.

Not all hearing-impaired individuals are binaural candidates. Some who have usable residual hearing in only one ear certainly cannot benefit from amplification in a dead ear. Others may show such a pronounced asymmetry in either their threshold pattern, suprathreshold distortions, or in speech discrimination skills that the second aid interferes with their perception through their good ear. If, however, in these instances, the addition of the second aid does not demonstrate any decrement in function, then a binaural aid should be tried. It is possible that some binaural superiority exists but is manifested only in a dimension difficult to objectively assess. (Because an auditory dimension is not or cannot be evaluated does not mean that such dimensions do not exist.) Also, for children who have never experienced binaural amplification, it frequently takes time for the auditory system to adjust before they can profit from the experience. This possibly may be related to a delay in exposure to a true binaural signal, which, when occurring, engages a unique population of auditory neurons. A lack of early stimulation of these fibers thus may preclude or limit binaural enhancement, making the adjustment difficult and prolonged. The clinical rule is, when in doubt, try.

CLASSROOM ACOUSTICS

Background noise

It is possible to provide early, functional, and properly adjusted hearing aids and yet still not ensure that the desired speech signal is clearly distinguishable from the background sounds. In our society, the environments in which verbal exchanges take place are noisy, and they appear to be getting more so. The rationale of an auditory approach, of employing amplified sound therapeutically for hearing-impaired children, requires a highly positive signal-to-noise ratio. This is a necessary precondition for linguistic development through an auditory mode.

What is not nearly well enough appreciated is that hearing-impaired persons are much more susceptible to the deleterious effects of noise than are normal hearing people. It is possible for a normal hearing person to communicate effectively in an unfavorable acoustic environment. It is extremely difficult for adventitiously hearing-impaired adults to do so, even given their normal background in speech and language development. It is almost impossible for young congenitally hearing-impaired children to develop their linguistic potential in such environments. Normal hearing persons and, less effectively, the adventitiously hearing-impaired adults can call on their normal knowledge of the language to fill the linguistic gaps for speech perception in unfavorable acoustic conditions (Fry, 1978; Ross, 1981b). The hearing-impaired child does not have this knowledge. This, indeed, is the major goal in employing amplification as a therapy tool.

Under normal classroom conditions, the average ratio between the teacher's voice and the background noise at the child's location is approximately 1 to five dB (Ross, 1978). Many classrooms present better conditions than this, but others show even more noise. In one recent survey of 45 classrooms, an average sound pressure level reading of 64 dB was found, with a standard deviation of 8 dB (Ross et al., 1982, p. 137). In one widely quoted study, normal hearing children shifted 35% in speech discrimination scores as the signal-to-noise ratio went from +12 dB to 0, whereas under the same conditions hard-of-hearing children's scores went from 83% to 39%, a shift of 46% (Finitzo-Hieber & Tillman, 1978). In terms of the optimal signal-to-noise ratio for the two populations, the hearing impaired required about 15 dB more signal to achieve their speech discrimination scores than the normal hearing (Leshowitz & Lindstrom, 1978). Considering the usual signal-to-noise conditions found in classrooms, this means that hearing-impaired children are precluded from the optimal use of their residual hearing in environments in which they are supposed to "listen and learn" from the teachers.

Reverberation

Reverberation is another kind of noise occurring in classrooms that is perhaps even more insidious and detrimental in its effects than general background noise. It has been defined as the repeated reflections of sound within an enclosure (Borrild, 1978). The more reverberant the room, the more the noise and the poorer the signal-to-noise ratio. It is as if every reflection of a direct sound is an additional source of sound, as indeed it is. Reverberation is insidious because a room may appear to be suitable until someone starts to talk. Then the reflections of some speech sounds overlap in time and mask later arriving speech sounds. Thus, in the word *off*, the reflection pattern of the strong vowel coexists with the later arriving /f/ and may render it inaudible or less audible.

Hearing-impaired people are more susceptible to the effects of reverberation than normal hearing people (Nabelek, 1980). In the study by Finitzo-Hieber and Tillman (1978), it was found that in quiet and at zero reverberation time, the speech discrimination scores for the normal hearing were 95% and for the hearing impaired, 83%. When the reverberation time increased to 1.2 sec, the scores for the normal hearing dropped to 77% (a decrease of 18%), whereas the scores for the hearing impaired dropped to 45% (a decrease of 38%). The study also showed that the situation is even worse when both noise and reverberation occur simultaneously, as is usually the case. The research in this area suggests that the optimal reverberation time for hearing-impaired children is between .3 to .4 sec, whereas normal hearing children can withstand reverberation times of .7 to .9 sec before speech comprehension is significantly disrupted (Borrild, 1978; Nabelek, 1980).

No matter how noisy or reverberant a room is, a child can usually be provided with a highly positive speech-to-noise ratio if the distance between the teacher's lips and the microphone of the hearing aid or auditory trainer is decreased. Every study that has ever investigated the effects of microphone–talker distance on speech comprehension has found that with each reduction of distance, speech discrimination scores increase (Ross, 1978). The explanation is simple. Given a constant background noise, say of 60 to 65 dB, the reduction of distance between the talker and the microphone increases the level of the speech, thus increasing the speech-to-noise ratio and consequently improving speech comprehension.

AUDITORY TRAINING SYSTEMS

The most efficient way to improve the level of the speech relative to the noise arriving at a child's ear is to employ an auditory training system that locates the microphone close to the teacher's mouth. All current auditory training systems are capable of doing this. In addition, however, such a system must (a) enable a child to auditorially self-monitor his or her own vocal output, (b) permit child-to-child communication through a child's personal microphone, (c) be electroacoustically adaptable for each individual child, and (d) allow for use variations within different educational settings. At the current time, a frequency modulation (fm) auditory training system meets all of these requirements and is the type recommended, particularly in regular school settings (Ross, 1981a).

There is no doubt that the use of an fm auditory training system in classrooms will improve a child's speech discrimination ability and thus enhance the comprehension of the teacher's lessons. Since the time of the first published study on the topic (Ross & Giolas, 1971), every study that has compared speech discrimination scores with personal hearing aids and fm systems has shown the same positive results (Ross, Giolas, & Carver, 1973; Setliff, 1975).

Every hearing-impaired child in regular schools should be considered a potential recipient of an fm auditory training system. Classrooms are noisy places, and hearing-impaired children are more prone to disturbances from poor acoustical conditions than normal hearing children. A properly adjusted and utilized fm system would ensure the full exploitation of the child's auditory potential. No other single therapeutic step can have the same powerful effect. If the notion is accepted that a child's learning in schools is related to how well the teacher can be heard and understood, then it follows that the more this ability can be improved, the more learning will occur. This does not imply that a program of language therapy is unnecessary, only that with an fm system the children can employ the linguistic competencies that they do possess to the fullest extent.

Not all educational situations lend themselves to fm systems. In an open-style classroom, where children are individually programmed for their learning activities and where little group work is done, such systems would be less effective. If communication with a teacher is always on a one-to-one basis, then in most instances it is possible for good auditory communication to take place, provided the teacher and the child are in close proximity. Most educational situations, however, usually combine individual and group lessons. The key principle in correctly using an fm system is for the teacher to ensure that the transmitter is turned on when it is intended that the child receive the transmission and turned off when the signal is inappropriate. Thus, when a child is a member of a class receiving instruction, the unit is turned on. When the child is doing seat work or is a member of a small group receiving instruction from a different teacher or aide, then the unit is turned off. (In this case, the other teacher should employ the unit.) This is one of the biggest problems in using fm systems in schools. Teachers frequently forget to turn the unit off when they should, and the child is then bombarded with several different signals simultaneously or receives unintended messages (such as when the principal enters the room to talk to the teacher about the child).

AUDITORY TRAINING

The following has little to do with what is traditionally called auditory training because the classic concept of auditory training is a last resort in therapy, to be applied logically and with rigor when necessary, but the need for which should have been precluded by application of the factors covered earlier. For the hard-of-hearing child in particular (i.e., the child who is potentially or is primarily dependent on the auditory channel for communication purposes), auditory training and speech and language development are one and the same (Ling, 1978b).

Exposure to language

Once the child is assured of receiving the highest fidelity amplified signal capable of being delivered, the same rules for linguistic growth apply as do for a normal hearing child. Hearing-impaired children possess a normal linguistic potential; from an auditory perspective, what they lack is a sufficient quantity and quality of relevant linguistic input. Attention to the factors already enumerated can ensure the quality, but this is not enough. The best amplified sound capable of being delivered is still being perceived in an impaired ear. It is certain that at least some acoustic information is missing and distorted. Fortunately, the acoustic spectrum of speech is highly redundant (Levitt, 1978). This redundancy, however, is more applicable for speech recognition than for linguistic development. To learn a language necessitates more of the acoustic information of speech than to recognize the same language once learned. Because the hearing loss reduces the amount and saliency of the speech signal, hearing-impaired children require a greater quantity of relevant linguistic inputs to compensate for this reduction in acoustic information (Fry, 1978). That is, to crack the linguistic code, they need much more exposure to it. Unlike normal hearing children, the language they hear (and overhear) is that directed specifically to them. They cannot hear what is going on in the next room, around the corner, or behind their backs. Thus, their exposure is limited, and they cannot as frequently make the desired associations with the nonlinguistic events related to the message.

Instead of receiving an enriched linguistic exposure, hearing-impaired children frequently receive less. Not only are they less aware of the linguistic events surrounding them, they may also receive less direct input because of their communicative difficulties. It takes a little more effort to talk to such children, and not everyone is willing to make the effort. This is not necessarily a conscious decision. Communication follows the path of the most reinforcement. If a hearing-impaired child does not appear to understand a specific message, then the language is simplified or gestures are substituted in order to attain comprehension. Once this mode has been established, a child who requires more exposure to the language winds up getting less. Many instances exist in which parents and teachers have consistently employed a simplified vocabulary and grammar so that comprehension could be ensured rather than expose the child to new words and structure, which require explication and slow down the communication process.

The implications of this observation are straightforward; children must be exposed much more to direct and relevant linguistic inputs. The language employed should be consistent with their cognitive level, interests, and activities, just as would be done with normal hearing children (Snow & Ferguson, 1977). A regime of "talk, talk, talk," which does not require or imply a response, is not being suggested but one of intensified conversation and discourse, in which two or more partners listen and converse. A child's utterance should be followed by expansions when necessary and a pertinent sequel (modeling). The goals are to engage children's natural capacity for linguistic development, perhaps the most powerful ally available in therapeutic endeavors with them and to provide them with enriching opportunities. Once they have been supplied with the maximum degree of relevant acoustic raw material, this intensified exposure to meaningful linguistic interchanges can be considered auditory training in a fundamental sense.

A structured approach

For many children, a natural auditory developmental model would not be sufficient. Some have found, for one reason or another, hearing to be an irrelevant, insufficient, or unstable avenue for communication purposes. Others attempt to employ audition as a primary communication mode but because of late and inadequate amplification or inadequate exposure have not reached their maximum capabilities. For these children, a more structured auditory training approach (i.e., a deliberate effort to enhance auditory capacities) is necessary. Several groups of children to whom this approach should be applied can be identified.

The first group of children consists of those who have found learning to be basically an irrelevant and probably unpleas-

---

The goals are to engage children's natural capacity for linguistic development, perhaps the most powerful ally available in therapeutic endeavors with them, and to provide them with enriching opportunities.

ant sensation. The use of audition was never emphasized in their training; few expectations were made regarding responses to sound, and little benefit seemed to accrue when auditory sensations were received. Thus, communicative and personal/social development took place without any significant contribution from the sense of hearing.

The first step with this group of children is to convince them that they can "hear" and that auditory sensations can confer advantages. Realistic limits have to be described and set for each child individually (since there are differences in the extent of their residual hearing). In a recent publication, possible procedures with these children and the groups of children described below have been outlined in detail (Ross et al., 1982).

The second group of children comprises those who employ hearing adequately in a complementary fashion with vision but are uncomfortable and insecure when presented with only auditory stimuli. As with the previous group, this group also needs confidence building, but starting from a higher level. Requiring responses from a known closed-set group of stimuli is a good place to begin. It is emphasized that the stimuli should be known to the children, since in these auditory-training tasks, the initial emphasis must be on the listening task and not language development. The closed set can be expanded in number or complexity, ensuring at each level that successful identification is possible. The children need the reinforcement of success. Tape-recorded paragraphs are a useful device, with the children having the written script in front of them from which predictable and then nonpredictable words and phrases are deleted. A telephone conversation is a motivating procedure for many of the older children. As training proceeds, the teacher can engage the children in relatively unstructured conversations or can present lesson material with his or her mouth covered. For these children, and at this stage, auditory training cannot only be a certain period set aside for that purpose; it must permeate the entire school day. The reciprocal relationship between speech and hearing must be explicitly emphasized throughout.

The final group of children consists of those who need refined discrimination training. Many hard-of-hearing children can begin their training at this level; others, such as the second group described above, can be brought up to it. Before proceeding with this stage, it is necessary to assess the children's speech discrimination ability, either through conventional word tests or through knowledge gleaned from therapeutic contacts with the children. Typically, this group of children will have difficulty identifying high-frequency consonants, particularly in the final position, as well as many unstressed morphological markers. In therapy, the phonemes and markers that they have difficulty perceiving are isolated, emphasized, and contrasted with other similar stimuli. Speech production training is an integral component of the training procedures at this stage, since it is known that assisting the child to produce a structure will reinforce its perception (Olmstead-Novelli, 1979). Auditory perception of many of these difficult sounds is difficult for many children; their degree and type of hearing loss may make it impossible for them to identify every phoneme and morphological marker. Fortunately, accoustical and linguistic redundancies supply the children with many alternative clues to perception. This possibility must be explained and demonstrated to them.

Speech reception

For all children in general, it must be recognized that in the reception of speech, the task is a search for the meaning of the utterances and not the identification of the specific constituent components. This is true not only for hearing-impaired children but for everyone. As people engage in conversation, they delve into the acoustic stream only as far as necessary to decode the message. If they need more information because of a particular ambiguity, they attend to the acoustic features necessary to resolve this ambiguity. Hearing-impaired children do the same thing. The problem is that they do not possess the same linguistic competencies that normal hearing people do, and thus they cannot as easily reconstruct the intended meaning of a message from the fragments they receive. The task of those working with the hearing impaired is twofold: One is to increase the linguistic store of the hearing impaired so as to optimize the central contribution to the perceptual process (Fry, 1978); the other is to increase the external information contained in the acoustic stream. This is called *auditory training*, but it cannot really be separated from linguistic competency in general.

It is in the reception process that the visual channel can make its greatest contribution for the hard-of-hearing children. Many of the acoustic features that are difficult for them to perceive are visually distinctive, and thus the combined mode can offer information to the total process of speech comprehension. The visual contribution was not emphasized because this article deals with amplification as a tool in linguistic development and because an emphasis on vision often seems to dominate the therapeutic process to the detriment of the full employment of the auditory channel. The visual channel is important, for some children vitally so, but for most hearing-impaired children it should be a supplemental and not a primary channel. Impaired or not, there is no more powerful channel for entering the biological capacities of children for learning speech and language than audition. For those who can profit from this approach—by no means all hearing-speech-language-impaired children—pathologists would be remiss in their professional responsibilities if they did not do all that they can to exploit the smallest fragment of residual hearing.

REFERENCES

Bendet, R.M. A public school hearing aid maintenance program. *Volta Review*, 1980, 82, 149–155.

Borrild, K. Classroom acoustics. In M. Ross & T.G. Giolas (Eds.), *Auditory management of hearing impaired children*. Baltimore: University Park Press, 1978.

Clopton, B.M., & Silverman, M.S. Plasticity of binaural

interaction: II. Critical period and changes in midline response. *Journal of Neurophysiology,* 1977, *40,* 1275–1280.

Danaher, E., & Pickett, J. Some masking effects produced by low frequencies vowel formants in persons with sensorineural hearing loss. *Journal of Speech and Hearing Research,* 1975, *18,* 261–271.

Dugal, R.L., Braida, L.D., & Durlach, N.I. Implications of previous research for the selection of frequency-gain characteristics. In G.A. Studebaker & I. Hochberg (Eds.), *Accoustical factors affecting hearing aid performance.* Baltimore: University Park Press, 1980.

Finitzo-Hieber, T., & Tillman, T.W. Room acoustics effects on monosyllabic word discrimination ability for normal and hearing-impaired children. *Journal of Speech and Hearing Research,* 1978, *21,* 440–458.

Fry, D.B. The role and primacy of the auditory channel in speech and language development. In M. Ross & T.G. Giolas (Eds.), *Auditory management of hearing-impaired children.* Baltimore: University Park Press, 1978.

Gaeth, J.H., & Lounsbury, E. Hearing aids and children in elementary schools. *Journal of Speech and Hearing Disorders,* 1966, *31,* 283–289.

Gottlieb, M.E., Zinkus, P.W., & Thompson, A. Chronic middle ear disease and auditory perceptual difficulty. *Clinical Pediatrics,* 1979, *18,* 725–732.

Kenker, F.J., McConnell, F., Logan, S.A., & Green, E.W. A field study of children's hearing aids in school environment. *Language, Speech, and Hearing Services in School,* 1979, *10,* 47–53.

Kessler, M., & Randolph, K. The effects of early middle ear disease on the auditory abilities of third grade children. *Journal of the Academy of Rehabilitative Audiology,* 1979, *12,* 6–20.

Killion, M.C. Earmold options for wideband hearing aids. *Journal of Speech and Hearing Disorders,* 1981, *46,* 10–20.

Leshowitz, B., & Lindstrom, R. Masking and speech-to-noise ratio. In D.O. McPherson (Ed.), *Proceedings of the Workshop on Prosthetics and Technical Devices for the Deaf.* Rochester, N.Y.: National Technical Institute for the Deaf, 1978.

Levitt, H. The acoustics of speech production. In M. Ross & T.G. Giolas (Eds.), *Auditory management of hearing impaired children.* Baltimore: University Park Press, 1978.

Libby, E.R. *Binaural hearing and amplification* (2 vols.). Chicago: Zenetron, 1980.

Libby, E.R., Johnson, J.H., & Longwell, T.F. *Innovative earmold coupling systems: Rationale, design, clinical applications.* Chicago: Zenetron, 1981.

Ling, D. Auditory coding and receding: An analysis of auditory training procedures for hearing-impaired children. In M. Ross & T.G. Giolas (Eds.), *Auditory management of hearing-impaired children.* Baltimore: University Park Press, 1978(a).

Ling, D. *Speech and the hearing-impaired child: Theory and practice.* Washington, D.C.: A.G. Bell Association, 1978(b).

Masters, L., & Marsh, G.E. Middle ear pathology as a factor in learning disabilities. *Journal of Learning Disorders,* 1978, *11,* 54–57.

Nabelek, A.K. Effects of room acoustics on speech perception through hearing aids by normal-hearing and hearing-impaired listeners. In G.A. Studebaker & I. Hochberg (Eds.), *Acoustical factors affecting hearing aid performance.* Baltimore: University Park Press, 1980.

Office of Demographic Studies. *Summary of selected characteristics of hearing impaired students* (Series D, No. 5). Washington, D.C.: Gallaudet College, 1971.

Olmstead-Novelli, T. *Production and reception of speech by hearing-impaired children.* Unpublished master's thesis, School of Communication Disorders, McGill University, Montreal, Canada, 1979.

Patchett, T.A. Auditory pattern discrimination in albino rats as a function of auditory restriction at different ages. *Developmental Psychology,* 1977, *13,* 168–169.

Pickett, J.M. *The sounds of speech communication.* Baltimore: University Park Press, 1980.

Ross, M. A review of studies on the incidence of hearing aid malfunctions. In, *The condition of hearing aids worn by children in a public school program* (HEW Publication No. (OE) 77–05002). Washington, D.C.: U.S. Government Printing Office, 1977.

Ross, M. Classroom acoustics and speech intelligibility. In J. Katz (Ed.), *Handbook of clinical audiology* (2nd ed.). Baltimore: Williams & Wilkins, 1978.

Ross, M. Binaural versus monaural hearing aid amplification for hearing impaired individuals. In E.R. Libby (Ed.), *Binaural hearing and amplification* (Vol. 2). Chicago: Zentron, 1980.

Ross, M. Classroom amplification. In W.R. Hodgson & P.H. Skinner (Eds.), *Hearing aid assessment and use in audiologic habilitation* (2nd ed.). Baltimore: Williams & Wilkins, 1981 (a).

Ross, M. Personal versus group amplification: The consistensy vs. inconsistency debate. In F. Bess (Ed.). *Amplification for education.* Washington, D.C.: A.G. Bell Association, 1981 (b).

Ross, M., Brackett, D., & Maxon, A.M. *Hard of hearing children in regular schools.* Englewood Cliffs, N.J.: Prentice-Hall, 1982.

Ross, M., & Giolas, T.G. Effect of three classroom listening conditions on speech intelligibility. *American Annals of the Deaf,* 1971, *116,* 580–584.

Ross, M., & Giolas, T.G. Introduction. In M. Ross & T.G. Giolas (Eds.), *Auditory management of hearing impaired children.* Baltimore: University Park Press, 1978.

Ross, M., Giolas, T.G., & Carver, P. Effect of three classroom listening conditions on speech intelligibility: A replication in part. *Language, Speech, and Hearing Services in School*, 1973, *4*, 72–76.

Setliff, W.M. *A study on hearing aid intelligibility in an acoustic preschool classroom.* Paper presented at the annual convention of the American Speech and Hearing Association, Washington, D.C., November 1975.

Snow, C.E., & Ferguson, C.S. *Talking to children: Language inputs and acquisition.* London: Cambridge University Press, 1977.

Studebaker, G.A., & Wark, D.J. *Factors affecting the intelligibility of hearing aid process speech.* Paper presented at the annual meeting of the American Speech-Language-Hearing Association, Detroit, November 1980.

Webster, D.B., & Webster, M. Neonatal sound deprivation affects brain stem auditory nuclei. *Archives of Otolaryngology*, 1977, *103*, 392–396.

Zinkus, P.W., & Gottlieb, M.I. Patterns of perceptual and academic deficits related to early chronic otitis media. *Pediatrics*, 1980, *66*, 246–253.

Language assessment protocols for hearing-impaired students

Diane Brackett, PhD
Assistant Professor
Communication Sciences
University of Connecticut
Storrs, Connecticut

TRADITIONALLY, language assessment of the hearing-impaired child in the public school has been the responsibility of public school personnel, whereas the evaluation of the hearing-impaired child in an outside placement has been left up to the private agency administering the program. In most cases, the outside evaluation consists of criterion-referenced testing on the skills that have been taught, rather than any norm-referenced tests, to determine the actual level at which the child is functioning. Criterion-referenced tests are adequate as long as the child remains in the same setting but they are inadequate when a determination for placement is to be made, since such a test does not provide a normative group against which the child can be compared. A few tests standardized on hearing-impaired children have been developed to establish levels of language competence. The Scales of Early Communication Skills for Hearing Impaired Children (Moog &

Geers, 1975) for children 2 to 9 years old and the Grammatical Analysis of Elicited Language Sentence Test (Moog & Geers, 1979) for children 2 to 8 years old were normed on hearing-impaired children. The Test of Syntactic Ability (Quigley, Steinkamp, & Power, 1978) has normative data on hearing-impaired children from 10 to 18 years of age.

Because the placement options for the hearing-impaired child have broadened to include different levels of mainstream education, the tests chosen must reflect the skills needed in these settings. Speech–language pathologists have long used tests standardized on normal hearing children to assess the communicative skills of the mildly impaired child in the public school, but little research exists on the use of these evaluation tools with more severely hearing-impaired children. Davis (1974) used the Boehm Test of Basic Concepts to demonstrate the difficulty that hearing-impaired children have in understanding verbal material. Geers and Moog (1978) compared the use of spontaneous language sampling with elicited language sampling for analyzing the productive language competency of hearing-impaired children.

Such studies do not indicate how to proceed in using test data for making placement decisions or designing remedial programs. Nor do they give needed information on criteria for evaluating the potential effectiveness of other assessment tools. In addition, children being educated in regular classrooms have not been regularly included in the subject pool.

The 1977 data gathered by the Office of Demographic Studies, Gallaudet College, reveal that 19% of the hearing-impaired people in the sample had received some or all of their education in the regular classroom (Karchmer & Trybus, 1977). One would expect even a larger number at the present time, since the impact of "least restrictive environment" has been felt. The hearing losses represented in this group ranged from mild to profound. One can assume that children with mild to moderate losses constitute the greatest portion of this group, since they traditionally have been the most frequently mainstreamed, most underserved, most ignored, and most undercounted, seemingly due to the less severe and obvious deficiencies they demonstrate. Nevertheless, children with varying degrees of hearing loss and ability to use the auditory channel are present in mainstream settings and demonstrate a range of communicative abilities, academic performance, and psychosocial skills (Reich, Hambleton, & Houldin, 1977). This heterogeneity makes it difficult to set up one set of language assessment protocols that is applicable to all children in all situations. By setting up methods of evaluating the communicative situation in which the child is asked to function and applying a set of criteria to evaluate the effectiveness of new assessment procedures, it is possible to design an evaluation that is pertinent to the needs of a particular child.

The purpose of the evaluation, either for determining placement or designing a remedial program, effects the selection of assessment tools. Certainly the impressions and recommendations would differ significantly depending on the stated purpose. If the ultimate goal is placement, the language evaluation must be considered in addition to other kinds of evaluations to

Table 1. Programming alternatives for hearing-impaired children

Title	Description of class	Peer group	Size	Communication demands
Segregated class	Special curriculum, housed in special education facility	Academic: hearing impaired; social: hearing impaired	Small class: 2 adults, 8 children	1. Use respond strategy rather than initiate. 2. Physically demonstrate rather than verbally explain. 3. Attend to adult input only. 4. Focus on producing spoken language, not on conversational skills. 5. Academic material geared to the child's language level and heavy reliance on visual aids. 6. Produce and comprehend written/read language at a level commensurate with hearing-impaired classmates.
Social mainstreaming	Regular classroom for art, music, gym, lunch, recess; all academics outside of regular class in resource room; special curriculum	Academic: hearing impaired; social: normal hearing, hearing impaired	Academic: small class; social: regular class, small class	1. Academic material is geared to the child's language level with heavy reliance on visual aids. 2. Produce and comprehend written/read language at a level commensurate with hearing-impaired classmates. 3. Produce and transmit a message during social interaction that is appropriate and intelligible.
Partial mainstreaming	Child enrolled in regular class for most of academic program; one or more of academic subjects in resource room; special curriculum for resource room subjects	Academic: normal hearing, hearing impaired; social: normal hearing	Academic: small class, regular class; social: regular class	1. Needs specific vocabulary to understand regular class academic material. 2. Comprehend complex syntax for directions. 3. Able to follow lecture format (if in regular class for lecture presentations). 4. Produce intelligible, well-formulated questions and answers for regular class participation. 5. Understand written/read language at a level commensurate with classmates. 6. Produce and transmit a message during social interaction that is appropriate and intelligible.

Table 1. Continued

Title	Description of class	Peer group	Size	Communication demands
Full mainstreaming	Child receives all academic subjects in the regular class; tutorial assistance is supplemental to the regular classroom curriculum.	Academic: normal hearing; social: normal hearing.	Academic: regular class; social: regular class.	1. Must be responsible for the language of all academic subjects. 2. Needs specific vocabulary to understand all academic material. 3. Comprehend syntax of spoken language for directions, social interaction, and teacher presentation. 4. Understand connected discourse. 5. Comprehend written/read language at a level commensurate with classmates. 6. Produce intelligible, well-formulated questions and answers for classroom participation. 7. Produce and transmit a message during social interaction that is appropriate and intelligible.

formulate a team decision as to the most appropriate setting for the child's education. If remedial programming is the ultimate goal, the language testing to be done serves to describe the child's strengths and weaknesses with goals for remediation of the deficit emerging from the description.

Not only does the purpose for the evaluation have a bearing on the selection of tests, but it also affects the skills to be evaluated. When evaluating the skills of a 5-year-old who has only recently been identified as hearing-impaired, the focus should be on determining the stage of language acquisition. When evaluating the skills of a 16-year-old who is being considered for a mainstreamed placement, the goal of the evaluation is not only to look at the child's communicative abilities as he or she interacts verbally with the environment but also how his or her language impacts on academic performance. Broadening the definition of language allows the child's interactive communicative abilities as well as his or her proficiency in receiving and using language in a graphic mode to be included.

A third factor that must be considered is the time available for the evaluation. The tests selected for an ongoing evaluation over a period of several weeks would be more extensive than if the evaluation were

Putting together pieces of information from a variety of standardized tests, language samples, and structured observation provides the most accurate description of the child's skills.

to take place during a 1½- to 2-hour period on a single day. It is critical to select those tools that will give the most information in the shortest amount of time if the time allotted for the evaluation is limited.

The availability of the tools is a fourth consideration. It is possible to make use of existing tests and adapt them to fit each child's needs rather than wait for the one definitive test that fits all of the criteria. Putting together pieces of information from a variety of standardized tests, language samples, and structured observation provides the most accurate description of the child's skills.

The fifth factor to consider is the availability of other information regarding the child's learning potential and achievement. An evaluation that synthesizes the language data with other areas of functioning allows for a more comprehensive description of the child's communicative set rather than just a reporting of his test performance. If the child has been diagnosed as having learning problems unrelated to the hearing loss, it is then possible to integrate the language results with the educational findings to formulate recommendations that take into account the child's optimal learning strategies.

If a placement decision is the ultimate goal, the communicative demands of the potential setting as well as previous setting must be considered as well as the expectations placed on the child within the setting. Some generalizations can be made about the level of communicative competence necessary to participate in each of the programming alternatives—segregated class, social mainstreaming, partial mainstreaming, and full mainstreaming.

Table 1 depicts these four programming alternatives and the communicative demands inherent in each.

The rationale for having these options available is that any one of them might be appropriate for a child at one time but not at another. Children must have the flexibility to adjust their communicative style to the new environment. If the children have always been mainstreamed, they are much less likely to have difficulty moving between these levels, since they have learned the social, communicative, and educational requirements. This does not hold true for children who are new to the mainstreamed setting, since they may be accustomed to the communicative set of a segregated or more protective setting. Frequently, the professionals responsible for suggesting such a placement change are not fully aware of the communicative adaptations necessary for making a successful adjustment in a more normalized setting. It is not uncommon to find that the professional's awareness of the children's deficits become diminished after a period of time. Their ears become accustomed to the poor quality of the speech and language. They begin to think that minor changes in the child's communicative status signal a need for a program change. Evaluations received from such personnel reflect this distorted view of communication. Observation of children in their previous placement and evaluation by an uninvolved professional could provide a more realistic view of their potential.

Aside from determining the communicative demands of the potential placement before the evaluation is done, consideration should be given to the expectations that accompany placing the child in the setting. The expectations may vary from social exposure to normal hearing children, exposure to academic material, partial learning of the academic material, or full participation as a member of a class.

Another reason to evaluate is to plan a remedial program based on the child's individual needs and to transmit the information to the professionals involved in educating the child. In the segregated class, special education teachers must be aware of the children's language status so they can gear their input to the children's level. In a mainstreamed setting, the regular classroom teacher, special teachers, and supportive personnel (tutor, reading consultant, social worker) need information on the way in which the child receives and produces spoken language. To carry out this essential part of the remedial program, the evaluation results must be reported in a manner that is accessible to the untrained or nonspecialized person.

Once the goals of the evaluation have been established, the actual assessment can be planned. The tools will consist of standardized tests, nonstandardized procedures, and structured observation of the child's communicative behavior in the educational context. No one test is adequate to describe a child's strengths and weaknesses. Frequently, professionals involved with hearing-impaired children are loath to use tests normed on normal hearing children, since the impaired child may perform badly on such tests. It is argued that the skills being tapped by these language tests are not visually or auditorally salient. English in its conversational form does lack readily accessible visual and auditory cues for all sounds and grammatical elements. But if the goal is to assess the reality of the situation, then it is necessary to measure the child's ability to deal with the language system.

An evaluation must be based on the skills that are needed to handle the communicative demands of a classroom. Examples of the complexities of classroom interactive language are as follows.

First grade: "Who can show us where we live? Who can show us where Connecticut is?" *Third grade:* "Who can tell us the story of what happens when you add three numbers together?" *Seventh grade:* "Now in that exercise, you had to pick out the adverb and tell what verb it modifies." *Tenth grade:* "If I say 'I'm waiting for,' do you want a direct object pronoun or an indirect?"

Even though the nature of the information being presented or elicited varies according to the academic level of the child, the complexity of the syntax and the specificity of the vocabulary remain remarkably consistent throughout. The children also require techniques for analyzing discourse, such as determining to whom or to what the pronoun refers in the previous clause or sentence. Comprehension of the words and syntax used in questions is essential, since a traditional teaching technique consists of eliciting information through a question/answer procedure. Comprehension of these features is complicated by the rate, loudness, and clarity of the actual presentation and the availability of visual input. These interactive language skills must be examined, and those skills necessary to understand and produce written language must be assessed as well. Written language increases in importance as academics are introduced throughout the grade levels. Underlying all of these skills is the ability of the child to receive the speech signal through visual, auditory, or combined modalities. The skills to be evaluated are summarized as follows:

1. Reception of spoken language
   PBK (phonetically balanced kindergarten) lists repeated after the clinician/teacher under three conditions: (a) look, (b) listen, (c) look and listen.
2. Comprehension of spoken language
   a. Single word receptive vocabulary: Peabody Picture Vocabulary Test, Test of Language Development (receptive vocabulary), Boehm Test of Basic Concepts
   b. Morphology and syntax: Test for Auditory Comprehension of Language, Northwestern Syntax Screening Test, Fullerton Test of Adolescent Language
   c. Paragraph comprehension: Durrell Paragraph Listening Test, Test of Auditory Comprehension (Subtests 8 and 10), Comprehensive Evaluation of Language Function
3. Production of spoken language
   a. Morphology and syntax
      i. Language sample analysis: Developmental Sentence Analysis (DSA), Kretschmer Spontaneous Language Analysis System
      ii. Elicited language sample: Carrow Elicited Language Inventory
      iii. Story completion: Story Completion Test; Structured Photographic Language Test
   b. Use
      i. Lexical: Wechsler Intelligence Scale for Children–Revised (WISC–R) (Vocabulary), Test of Language Development (Oral Vocabulary), Detroit Test of Learning Aptitude (Verbal Opposites, Likenesses and Differences), Fullerton Test of Adolescent Language (Homonyms)
      ii. Connected speech: Detroit Test of Learning Aptitude (Verbal Absurdities, Social Adjustment A), WISC–R (Information, Comprehension)
4. Comprehension and production of written language
   a. Comprehension of written syntax: Test of Syntactic Abilities
   b. Production: Test of Written Language, Written Language Sample
5. Production of speech
   a. Sound and syllable level: Phonetic and Phonological Evaluation (Ling, 1976).
   b. Word level: Standard Articulation Test, Phonetic and Phonological Evaluation (Ling, 1976).
   c. Speech production intelligibility: NTID Rating Scale, Sentences for Assessment of Speech Production Intelligibility (Seewald, 1981).
6. Communicative competence
   a. Function of language: sustains topic of conversation, flexible lan-

guage system, politeness and authoritarian routines present, adapts message after communication failure or on listener request (Simon, 1981).
b. Style of language use: aware of listener's knowledge and status by adapting the message, conversational turn taking, and entry points (Simon, 1981).

The language delay exhibited by most hearing-impaired children makes it necessary to use standardized tests normed on much younger normal hearing children. For example, it is not uncommon to use a test normed on normal hearing children from 3 years 0 months to 6 years 11 months when evaluating the language status of a preadolescent hearing-impaired child. The score obtained has a function in that it demonstrates how severely delayed the child is in comparison to his or her normal hearing peers. If placement decisions must be made, based partially on the communication evaluation, then the designation of a language level would be beneficial. The score or scores by themselves do not provide the kind of information necessary to design and implement a remedial program for a hearing-impaired child. Rather, a more purposeful use of these tests is to describe the abilities of the child. This description should include information regarding the nature of the communication deficit and the circumstances under which communication failure occurs. Performance on a specific test should not be limited to a test score; it should provide an account of children's linguistic deficits and abilities, their test-taking strategies, and a prediction as to the impact of the communication problem on nontest interactions (Ross, Brackett, & Maxon, 1982).

Test presentation must take into account the fact that the child has a hearing loss. Therefore, the first step in any evaluation is to ensure that the child's amplification is functioning properly. If the test requires a face-to-face presentation, then care must be taken to make the visual information available. The results of the assessment can then be interpreted to represent the child's optimal performance when he or she is receiving maximum auditory and visual information (Davis & Hardick, 1981).

To avoid penalizing the child, it may be necessary to modify the standardized procedure by presenting the stimulus items several times, with the additional option of having the child repeat what he or she has heard. Adding a written representation of a verbal stimulus should be done with caution, since it may somewhat alter the purpose of using a specific test. For example, if the purpose of using a paragraph comprehension test is to assess the child's ability to understand connected discourse in its spoken form, then pairing the spoken stimulus with a written translation would significantly change the interpretation of the result. The information regarding the child's ability to cope with a lecture format in a classroom would no longer be available from the test.

Interpretation of the test results should be made in light of the interaction between the child's auditory status and his or her test performance. A distinction can be made between those responses resulting from deficiencies in the child's linguistic system as opposed to those errors resulting

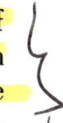

> *It is only through testing the evaluation results against more informal communicative observations that a functional diagnosis can be made.*

from difficulty with the reception of the stimuli. Is the child able to hear /s/ when it marks the plural (as in *coats*), or does he or she hear the /s/ but not understand the meaning contained in the /s/ phoneme when used as a plural marker? The child's response to the stimuli appears the same regardless of the reason, but remedial techniques vary greatly (Ross, Brackett, & Houldin, 1982).

The way in which the language deficit is translated into reality becomes critical when the evaluation information is transmitted to personnel directly involved with the hearing-impaired child. It is not uncommon to find that the child's errors are task related or test dependent and may not be demonstrated in real situations. The reverse situation, in which the child's test performance overestimates his or her actual ability, also occurs. It is only through testing the evaluation results against more informal communicative observations that a functional diagnosis can be made. This final step in the evaluation process requires the examiner to observe the child as he or she interacts in a classroom setting. The five areas of classroom behavior in which the child's communicative abilities have the most impact are

- participation in classroom activities and discussion
- interaction between the child and teacher, both verbal and social
- interaction between the child and peers, both verbal and social
- strategies the child demonstrates for learning content material presented in a lecture format
- adaptations made by the teacher of the orally presented material.

INTERPRETATION

The results of tests that assess similar areas of language can be grouped when their impact on classroom behavior is being considered. For example, all of the tests that assess the understanding of spoken language (Peabody Picture Vocabulary Test, Test for Auditory Comprehension of Language, Durrell, Boehm) have a similar effect on the child's performance in the classroom. Some typical behaviors resulting from deficient verbal comprehension might be difficulty with (a) content material presented in a lecture format, (b) language-based subjects (reading, science, social studies), (c) understanding interactive classroom language (specifically questions, instructions, and classroom discussion), and (d) attending during verbal presentations. The modifications for a child who demonstrates a deficiency in verbal comprehension might include (a) using visual support such as writing on the blackboard or overhead projector, (b) using a hands-on demonstration of the material, (c) giving the child an outline of the lesson prior to class, (d) previewing the vocabulary and concepts by the tutor, (e) paraphrasing the lecture material by using less complex syntax and vocabulary, and (f) questioning the child's understanding through content questions.

The assessment results can also be used to design a remedial program. Depending on the educational setting in which the child is placed, the level of direct service that the child receives from the speech–language pathologist varies. If the child is in a segregated class, the description of the child's strengths and weaknesses provides the classroom teacher with the information needed for planning the language curriculum in the classroom. The child might also receive intensive service from the speech–language pathologist. Both professionals would be attempting to improve the child's language skills. For example, using the grouped results of the verbal comprehension tests, the classroom teacher and the speech–language pathologist might select a similar goal (i.e., understanding the past tense endings) and work on it in individual and group sessions. In a mainstreamed setting, the teacher needs to be aware of the child's language limitations to make classroom modifications but may not spend time remediating the deficit area. Rather, it becomes the speech–language pathologist's responsibility to provide direct intervention. If the child displayed a deficit in understanding the vocabulary related to directions, the speech–language pathologist would work directly on the lexical items, whereas the regular classroom teacher would try to modify the verbal and written instructions so that the child could participate in the activity.

By grouping the results according to the skill measured, it is possible to project a broader picture of the child's communication system and the ultimate impact of the educational process. The same approach can be applied to other deficit areas that emerge.

• • •

Protocols chosen to evaluate the communication skills of hearing-impaired children must reflect the purpose and time alloted of the evaluation, age of the child, availability of tests, and the impact of other information concerning their learning abilities. Standardized tools and structured observation of the children as they function in a verbal environment should be used to assess the children's skills. Skills proficiency should be matched with the communicative demands of the educational setting to make programming decisions and determine remedial goals.

REFERENCES

Davis, J. Performance of young hearing impaired children on a test of basic concepts. *Journal of Speech and Hearing Research*, 1974, *17*, 342–351.

Davis, J., & Hardick, E. *Rehabilitative audiology for children and adults*. New York: Wiley, 1981.

Geers, A., & Moog, J. Syntactic maturity of spontaneous speech and elicited imitations of hearing impaired children. *Journal of Speech and Hearing Disorders*, 1978, *43*, 380–391.

Karchmer, M.A., & Trybus, R.J. *Who are the deaf children in mainstream programs?* (Series R, No. 4) Washington, D.C.: Office of Demographic Studies, 1977.

Ling, D. *Speech and the hearing-impaired child: Theory and practice*. Washington, D.C.: A.G. Bell Association, 1976.

Moog, J.S., & Geers, A. *Grammatical analysis of elicited language*. St. Louis: Central Institute for the Deaf, 1979.

Moog, J.S., & Geers, A. *Scales of early communication skills for hearing impaired children.* St. Louis: Central Institute for the Deaf, 1975.

Quigley, S.P., Steinkamp, M.W., & Power, D.J. *Test of syntactic abilities.* Beaverton, Ore.: Dormac, 1978.

Reich, C., Hambleton, D., & Houldin, B. The integration of hearing impaired children in regular classrooms. *American Annals of the Deaf,* 1977, *122,* 534–544.

Ross, M., Brackett, D., & Maxon, A. *Hard of hearing children in the regular classroom.* Englewood Cliffs, N.J.: Prentice-Hall, 1982.

Seewald, R. *The interrelationships among hearing loss utilization of auditory and visual cues in speech reception and speech production intelligibility in children.* Unpublished doctoral dissertation, University of Connecticut, Storrs, 1981.

Simon, C. *Communicative competence: A functional-pragmatic approach to language therapy.* Tucson, Ariz.: Communication Skill Builders, 1981.

Language intervention for hearing-impaired children from linguistically and culturally diverse backgrounds

Joseph E. Fischgrund, MA
Director
Projecto Opportunidad
Rhode Island School for the Deaf and Brown University
Providence, Rhode Island

THE PRINCIPAL of the Rhode Island School for the Deaf received an inquiry in 1921 from a Brown University professor of the social sciences inquiring about the children of foreign-born families then in attendance at the School for the Deaf. After citing numbers indicating that over half of the schoolchildren had parents who did not speak English, the principal added the following comment: "In families of foreign parentage I find the progress in speech and language much retarded—when the pupils are at their homes from the fact that if the parents speak English it is 'broken English,' hard to interpret by people with all their faculties, and particularly puzzling for a speech or lip reader" (Hurd, 1921). Unfortunately, the observation that deaf children from non-English-speaking (NES) homes face additional difficulties in school was to go virtually unnoticed in deaf education for over half a century.

In 1976, responding to the increasing

number of Hispanic students in programs for the hearing impaired in New York City, Lerman (1976) conducted an extensive survey of hearing-impaired students in that area. He noted that "a disproportionate number [of Hispanic students] are placed in the low achieving or learning disabled groups in the schools" (p. 1). Lerman also cited data from Jensema (1975) establishing that "Spanish-American deaf students have lower achievement levels than white deaf students and, in vocabulary and reading comprehension, lower levels than other minority groups surveyed" (p. 10).

Responding to a growing national awareness of the difficulties that hearing impaired students from NES homes were encountering in school, Delgado (1981) conducted the first thorough national study of hearing-impaired students from NES homes. The number of these students nationally was reflective of the overall population of Hispanics and other NES groups, but the placement of students within programs for the hearing impaired was dramatically different. Whereas 29% of all students in programs for the hearing impaired were reported to have handicapping conditions in addition to hearing impairment, 51% of the students from NES homes were reported to have additional handicapping conditions. In the categories of mental retardation, emotional or behavioral disorder, and specific learning disability, three to four times as many hearing-impaired students from NES homes were said to have one of those additional disabilities as were students in the general hearing-impaired population. More significant, however, were the attitudes that Delagado found; for example,

"one large southwestern program for the deaf reported that only two children came from such a setting. The state involved has a very high Hispanic population. This response is a graphic indication of a prevalent and growing problem in the United States, and one that generally has been ignored" (p. 118).

Responding to changes in its own population, the Rhode Island School for the Deaf initiated bilingual/bicultural services in 1975. The program has resulted in lower dropout rates, better attendance, increased parent participation, and, a surprising side effect, a greater degree of mainstreaming for students from NES homes. In developing such a program, it is important to address the complex linguistic, sociolinguistic, and cultural issues inherent in developing a bilingual/bicultural program for linguistically and culturally diverse hearing-impaired children.

LINGUISTIC CONSIDERATIONS

The most immediate response to bilingual programming for hearing-impaired students is that since it is so hard for the deaf child to learn one language, how can the child be burdened with the task of learning two? This question is unwarranted for several reasons, most of which center around the conditions under which first and second languages are acquired.

First, the hearing-impaired child does not have a choice when it comes to the oral language environment of his or her home. Since exposure to language is the first step in language development, hearing-impaired children entering educational programs, no matter how severe their

> *The child has already been exposed to one language and will continue to be exposed to that language as long as it is the language of the home.*

hearing loss, have already begun the process of language acquisition. This position implies the rejection of descriptions of children, concluding that they have no language and an acceptance of a view of language as more than just an inventory of producible phonemes or testable vocabulary (e.g., Halliday, 1974). Whatever the language competence of the child, even if it is at the level of preverbal linguistic functioning, it is in the language of the home. This obviously follows from the maxim that the child acquires only that language that he or she is exposed to. Bolen (1981) suggested that "if the child has a severe-to-profound hearing loss ... from a linguistic point of view the educational process would be facilitated if the child were exposed to only one language (p. 411). What Bolen fails to account for is that the child has already been exposed to one language and will continue to be exposed to that language as long as it is the language of the home. Contrary to Bolen's position, it is contended here that this early exposure to the home language must be accounted for in the child's early educational program and that his or her continued exposure to the home language must be taken into account throughout the child's educational career.

Many hearing-impaired students, especially those with less than profound losses, do have demonstrable abilities in their native language when they enter the American (mainland) educational system. This range of abilities needs to be assessed along two parameters: the level of ability in the first language and the degree of bilingualism, if any. The nature of linguistic abilities that the child enters school with along these two parameters is probably the critical factor in educational success for children with significant degrees of residual hearing. As Bolen (1981) notes: "If the child has a mild, moderate, or moderate-to-severe hearing loss, there appears to be no reason why he or she cannot be bilingual from the start (p. 411).

Historically, programs for hearing-impaired students from NES homes have been designed for their hearing impairment but not for their underlying language abilities. For example, the moderately hearing-impaired adolescent with demonstrable proficiency in Spanish will generally be placed with students of his or her age level who have the lowest degree of English functioning or in a life skills or other program for low-functioning deaf students. If the program is in a school for the deaf, the student most likely will be placed with students with a far greater degree of hearing loss or with students whose problems in the acquisition of English are different. For example, in his study of New York City schools for the deaf, Lerman (1976) found significant differences in the age of onset category, "where 30% of all Hispanic students are reported as becoming deaf after birth, compared to 22% of the 'white' population" (p. 3).

For hearing-impaired students from

NES homes to have equal access to the specially designed services available to other hearing-impaired individuals, they need to have access to the language of that education—English. Conversely, programs for the hearing impaired need to adapt to the language abilities of the students as they enter the program. If there are educationally adequate abilities in the first language, then educational progress can continue in the home language while English is being acquired as a second language. For the hearing-impaired child whose language abilities are delayed in the first language because of the presence of the impairment, the optimal conditions under which the child will begin to enter into a second language-learning process is if there is continued development and use of the first language.

The support for this approach, for both hearing and hearing-impaired children, is found in the developmental interdependence hypothesis (Cummins, 1979). This hypothesis proposes that "the level of L2 [the second language] competence which a bilingual child attains is partially a function of the type of competence the child has developed in L1 [the first language] at the time when intensive exposure to L2 begins" (p. 222). Without attention to this linguistic interdependence, most hearing-impaired children find themselves in the situation described by Cummins: "If in an early stage of its development a minority child finds itself in a foreign-language learning environment without contemporaneously receiving the requisite support in its mother tongue, the development of its skill in the mother tongue will slow down and even cease, leaving the child without a basis for learning the second language (Cummins, 1979, p. 233). This situation, the most common one for most hearing-impaired children at all levels of hearing loss, explains the two most common complaints about hearing-impaired children from NES homes: complaints from the parents that the child is losing his or her home language and complaints from the teacher that the child is not doing well in school. Rather than explain these difficulties by saying, in the first case, that the child would rather speak English or, in the second case, that the child has an additional disability, one only has to look to the developmental interdependence hypothesis to understand why communication breakdown in the home and poor academic achievement are interrelated.

Acquiring a language and learning through language are two very different tasks. For the second to even become a possibility, the first, the process of language acquisition, must not only be happening but must have reached a certain threshold level. According to Cummins (1979), "there may be threshold levels of linguistic competence which a bilingual child must attain both in order to avoid cognitive disadvantages and allow the potentially beneficial aspects of bilingualism to influence his or her cognitive and academic functioning" (p. 222). This predicts that the child whose greater competence is in the home language but is asked to learn in English will not only suffer a cognitive disadvantage in the learning process but that whatever potential benefits are to be had from the child's abilities in his or her first language will be dissipated. For the child who has a hearing impairment, this principle, which involves the central role that language plays in the educational process, is of utmost importance not only in explaining the difficulties that hearing-impaired children from NES homes have experienced to date but also in developing language and educational programs that utilize all of the student's language abilities and do not place him or her at a cognitive disadvantage relative to his or her hearing-impaired peers.

This mismatch between home and school languages is not only a matter of the school's language being English and the child's home's language being other than English. The function of language in school and the form that it takes are unlike the form and function of language in the home. As Halliday (1974) notes: "The child who does not succeed in the school system may be one who is not using language in the ways required by the school" (p. 18) and that the failure of a student to master school skills is part of a more general problem, "the fundamental mismatch between the child's linguistic capabilities and the demands that are made upon them" (p. 18). The mismatch is more than just a consequence of the school and home languages' having different surface structures; it is a mismatch between the ways that languages are used at home and the way language is used in school. Halliday (1974) focuses on three areas of language functioning—the interpersonal (with properties arising from its use in social interaction), the ideational (which involves the use of language in conceptual learning), and the textual (with properties arising from the structure of the language itself), and points to aspects of the ideational area as "crucial to success in school" (p. 18).

For children from NES homes, Cummins (1981) points out the mismatch between the function of language at home and at school in terms of the language's being either context-embedded or context-reduced. According to Cummins, "context-embedded communication is more typical of the everyday world outside the classroom, whereas many of the linguistic demands of the classroom reflect communication which is closer to the context-reduced end of the continuum" (p. 34). With hearing-impaired students, as with students who are both hearing and hearing impaired from NES homes, an adequate level of interpersonal or context-embedded language and speech often mislead educators into thinking that the child is ready to learn in school when in fact the child may not have mastered the ideational function of language and thus cannot handle the context-reduced language environment of the school. When working with hearing-impaired children from NES homes, it is important not only to assess whether the child has the surface fluency in the linguistic system of the school but also whether the child has the range of functions in language, both in the home and school languages, that will allow him or her to successfully function in school. In terms of developing a program for hearing-impaired children from NES homes, Halliday's (1974) suggestion, intended for hearing students from English-speaking homes, for language education in general provides a useful guideline: "A minimum requirement for an educationally relevant approach to language is that it takes account of the child's own linguistic experience, defining this experience in terms of its richest potential and noting where there may be differences of orientation which could cause certain children difficulties in school" (p. 19).

The linguistic issues surrounding the education of linguistically and culturally diverse hearing-impaired students are not simple, and solutions to their educational and communicative problems likewise will not be simple. Only by taking into account their prior linguistic experience and abilities, by recognizing the role of these experiences in their cognitive and second language growth, and by recognizing the complexity of language functioning in school can one begin to appropriately assess and educate hearing-impaired students from linguistically and culturally diverse backgrounds.

LANGUAGE ASSESSMENT

The first task for the educator or clinician in preparing for language and educational intervention with the hearing-impaired child from an NES home is the task of language assessment. To appropriately evaluate the child's language ability, one must first ask the general question, What is the nature of the thing to be tested? (For a general discussion of bilingual assessment, see Erickson & Omark, 1981.) In potential bilingual situations, the key areas of assessment are language dominance and language proficiency. Hernandez-Chavez, Burt, and Dulay (1978), in an article on language dominance and proficiency testing, noted that three parameters of language proficiency need to be examined: linguistic components, modality, and sociolinguistic performance. Because the child has a hearing impairment and usually an associated language delay, the level of the language that the child has reached must also be assessed. It is important to differentiate between developmental level and proficiency, with the former being a description of the language itself and the latter an assessment of how those language abilities are used.

Given that developmental level, language dominance, and proficiency in whatever language systems exist need to be assessed, the choices of where and how to start and what instruments to use become far less difficult than they may initially appear. First, since one is looking at a broad range of language abilities, there is no need for the use of so-called psycholinguistic assessment instruments. Use of these instruments is a questionable practice for hearing-impaired children in general, since it has not been established that the specific abilities tested are those that underlie language acquisition (cf. Bloom & Lahey, 1978). Use with children from other cultures is even more questionable, since it is not at all clear that the form of the task itself is within the child's experience. This is especially true of recent immigrant children whose unfamiliarity with the task produces such low performance levels that they are often mislabled on the basis of inappropriate measures. In addition, these instruments, which are said to be nonverbal but in practice are not, do utilize language, and thus the child's prior language experience may be ignored or in direct contrast with the language of the test.

In focusing on language itself, rather than processing type tasks, it is also important to specify which aspects of the child's linguistic performance are most indicative of the developmental level of the child's language and are most useful in determining dominance or proficiency. Vocabulary testing, even in translation, is not an adequate linguistic measure, nor should it be used to indicate mental age in assessing hearing-impaired children from other cultures and language backgrounds. Vocabulary reflects the cultural and educational level of a speaker, not his or her linguistic level. In terms of the linguistic components that are meaningful in language assessment, Hernandez-Chavez et al. (1978) noted that "grammar—the morphology and syntax—are the best understood in terms of developmental processes, and, at least for the present, provides the most adequate research and methodological basis for making judgement about levels of language proficiency" (p. 51). A growing body of knowledge in semantics and pragmatics also allows us to add those areas to the list of linguistic components that are important to assess.

Depending on the child's background—recency of arrival, language status of the home (monolingual or bilingual), previous educational experience—the choice is made whether to assess developmental level or dominance first. If the child is a recent immigrant and from a totally NES home, then the question of dominance is a clear one, for surely there is no acquisition of English without exposure to it. If the child is from a bilingual background or has had some schooling in English, then dominance might be addressed first.

Dominance essentially is the question of which is the child's stronger language, and dominance testing must take into account how the child's abilities compare across language domains. It is not uncommon, for example, to find that hearing-impaired students with severe losses are dominant in different domains. Because most of their education has been in English, their dominant language for learning is English. However, when one considers the fluency and intelligibility of their speech, and especially in the area of suprasegmental phonology, they are clearly not dominant in English in the interpersonal function of language. Older hearing-impaired children are often more proficient in context-embedded (interpersonal) language in the home language but, because of prior educational experience, more proficient in context-reduced (ideational) language in English. On the other hand, many young (3- to 5-year-old) children with a moderate hearing impairment who come from bilingual homes often indicate a level of context-embedded social language in English that misleads educators and evaluators into thinking that the children are ready to function in school in English when that is really not the case. These relative abilities should not be seen as conflicting but rather as strengths that can be utilized in the student's educational development.

Assessment of the child's developmental level in language should be a descriptive one in the case of all hearing-impaired children, and a hearing-impaired child from an NES home presents only a variation of the same process that would be

---

It is not uncommon to find that hearing-impaired students with severe losses are dominant in different domains.

used to do a descriptive language evaluation of any other hearing-impaired child. Blackwell, Engen, Fischgrund, and Zarcadoolas (1978) argued convincingly that the use of normative data in language assessments of hearing-impaired students is of minimal interest and utility in developing and placing students in an appropriate language education program or in presenting a framework for describing the language of hearing-impaired children. This approach focuses on what the children have developed instead of attempting to find deficits in the child's language. The latter approach often leads to programming through a deficit model, which seeks to address aspects of the child's language performance that are said to be deviant rather than to provide an overall context for language structures and functions that have not yet been acquired or developed.

In general, assessment of the limited English proficient hearing-impaired child should include an elicited and spontaneous sample of the child's productive language in both home language and English, with all materials used for elicitation being similar but culturally appropriate. A comparable measure of comprehension should be used in both languages so that receptive abilities can be both assessed in the individual languages and compared to ascertain dominance and relative proficiency (cf. Engen & Engen, in press). Assessing the linguistic abilities that a child does have, as opposed to the aspects of English the child does not know, is the first step in the appropriate assessment of hearing-impaired students from linguistically and culturally diverse backgrounds.

CULTURAL CONSIDERATIONS

The NES child, no matter how profound the hearing impairment, brings his or her home culture to school, and it is not something that is turned off or on by leaving one door and entering another. A major aspect, and often the first encountered, is the family's view of the handicapping condition of the child and the demands that education places on its members in addition to the presence of the child. For many Hispanic families, for example, the handicap of the child can be dealt with in the context of their own community, religious orientation, and belief system, but what they cannot handle are the ways in which the school expects them to participate in the child's educational program. For the typical caretaker of the Puerto Rican hearing-impaired child (Lerman, 1976), the school or clinic can be an imposing, unapproachable institution, despite the best intentions of the professionals there. An active, culturally appropriate parent involvement program is a necessary component of any bilingual/bicultural program for hearing-impaired children if parental understanding, cooperation, and support are to be expected. The culturally diverse parent is not a parent who does not care, but is most often a parent who simply does not understand what is being asked of him or her.

A major task for hearing-impaired children is that of coming to terms with the culture of their home and that of their school and peers. Rather than assuming that the child is confused and thus should only be presented with one cultural (and linguistic) model, Blackwell and Fischgrund (in preparation) argue that the problem facing the hearing-impaired child is that he or she does not have enough conceptual data to understand the differences between the home and school cultures and his or her own place as a developing bicultural person. School curricula generally focus on information that is said to be central to the mainstream of American culture, but for the child who does not have an early grasp of what that mainstream is, there is no conceptual framework with which to assimilate new information. As a result, the child is often placed in a position of knowing only that something is different and, with some unintentional but powerful peer influence, often concludes that what is different, namely, his or her parents and home life, is inferior. For the hearing-impaired child from a cultural background different from the school's to come to terms with a bicultural environment, there needs to be a meaningful organization of information. This is the goal of a bicultural curriculum.

Overlapping the purely cultural conditions are the socioeconomic difficulties in which many non-English-speaking families find themselves. The families' priorities are a function of their social and economic status. If they are poor, newly arrived immigrants, one can be sure that regular visits to the otologist, hearing aids, or individualized educational plan (IEP) meetings are not high on the priority list, especially in the light of realities like food, clothing, and adequate shelter. In their desire to begin intervention relative to the child's handicap, special education program staff often assume that the families' priorities in other areas are the same or, if problematical, not the school's business.

Lerman and Fischgrund (1980) argued that "working with children from poor, immigrant families requires a new role for the school" (p. 10) and that the view that "limits the school's responsibilities to the activities of the children to the school day . . . leads to large numbers of dropouts and unserved children" (p. 10).

CHALLENGES IN EDUCATION

Cultural pluralism still appears to be a fact of American life, and despite an overall impression that the massive immigration of the early 20th century is over, much cultural and linguistic diversity is still present in America today. This is of course reflected in educational institutions and no less in educational programs for the hearing impaired.

Language also appears to be the critical factor in educating all children from culturally and linguistically diverse homes and is no less critical in programs for the hearing impaired. For these children to have equal access to educational opportunity, programs addressing the issues outlined in the preceding pages need to be developed. One such program is Projecto Oportunidad, the bilingual/bicultural program at the Rhode Island School for the Deaf. Other programs for the hearing impaired are currently being developed. Careful attention in these programs to the complex linguistic and sensitive cultural issues involved provides hope that the depressed achievement levels of hearing-impaired students from NES homes (Delgado, 1981; Jensema, 1975; Lerman, 1976) is a situation that will not exist in the near future.

It has long been a guiding proposition in bilingual/bicultural education that the child's home language and culture can be either a positive or negative factor in the child's education, but is is never neutral. Certainly no educator wishes to promote a negative factor, and attempts to neutralize by ignoring the child's home language and culture are doomed to fail. The challenge, then, for educators of hearing-impaired children from culturally and linguistically diverse homes is to utilize that cultural and linguistic richness in the most positive fashion, for the benefit of those particular students and their families and for all hearing-impaired students.

REFERENCES

Bolen, D. Issues relating to language choice—Hearing impaired infants from bilingual homes. *Volta Review,* 1981, *83,* 410–412.

Blackwell, P., Engen, E., Fischgrund, J., & Zarcadoolas, C. *Sentences and other systems: A language and learning curriculum for hearing impaired students.* Washington, D.C.: A.G. Bell Association of the Deaf, 1978.

Blackwell, P., & Fischgrund, J. A rationale for bilingual/bicultural programming for hearing impaired students. In G. Delgado (Ed.), *The hispanic deaf: Issues and challenges.* Book in preparation, 1982.

Bloom, L., & Lahey, M. *Language development and language disorders.* New York: Wiley, 1978.

Cummins, J. Linguistic interdependence and the educational development of bilingual children. *Review of Educational Research,* 1979, *49,* 222–251.

Cummins, J. Four misconceptions about language proficiency in bilingual education. *NABE Journal,* 1981, *5*(3), 31–45.

Delgado, G. Hearing impaired children from non-native language homes. *American Annals of the Deaf,* 1981, *126*(2), 118–121.

Engen, E., & Engen, T. *Test of language comprehension.* Baltimore, Md.: University Park Press, in press.

Erickson, J., & Omark, D. *Communication assessment of the bilingual bicultural child.* Baltimore, Md.: University Park Press, 1981.

Halliday, M. A. K. *Explorations in the functions of language.* London: Edward Arnold, 1974.

Hernandez-Chavez, E., Burt, M., & Daly, H. Language dominance and proficiency testing: Some general considerations. *NABE Journal,* 1978, *3*(1), 41–54.

Hurd, A. *Letter to Harold S. Bucklin.* Providence: Rhode Island School for the Deaf Archives, May 3, 1921.

Jensema, C. *The relationship between academic achievement and the demographic characteristics of hearing impaired youth.* Washington, D.C.: Gallaudet College, Office of Demographic Studies, 1975.

Lerman, A. *Discovering and meeting the needs of hispanic hearing impaired children* (Final Report, CREED VII Project). New York: Lexington School for the Deaf, 1976.

Lerman, A., & Fischgrund, J. *Improving services to hispanic hearing impaired students and their families.* Paper presented at the 9th annual meeting of NABE, Anaheim, California, April 1980.

Assessing language in young deaf adults

Gerard G. Walter, EdD
Chairperson
Department of Communication
  Assessment
  and Advising
National Technical Institute
  for the Deaf
Rochester, New York

C. Tane Akamatsu, PhD
Assessment and Advising
  Specialist/Language
Department of Communication
  Assessment
  and Advising
National Technical Institute
  for the Deaf
Rochester, New York

A SEVERE TO profound impairment in the auditory mechanism makes the learning of English (or any other auditorily based language) a monumental task for the afflicted individual. Cooper and Rosenstein (1966), Moores (1970), Swisher (1976), and Trybus and Karchmer (1977) have reported on English skills of persons with severe to profound hearing loss. They all come to the same conclusion: In reading, in writing, and in speaking, deaf individuals lag significantly behind their hearing peers. Some studies comparing the psycholinguistic abilities of deaf and hearing individuals have concluded that deaf persons may not only exhibit retardation in English development, but may be using rules to process English that are different from the rules used by their hearing peers (Bochner, 1978; Moores, 1971; Sarachan-Deily & Love, 1974; Tweeny & Hoemann, 1973).

Given the deficit in development of English skills referenced above and the characterization by Schlesinger and Meadow (1971) of deafness as more than a communication handicap—as a "cultural phenomenon in which social, emotional, linguistic and intellectual patterns and problems are inextricably bound together" (p. 1)—it is not surprising that deaf people, by virtue of their isolation from the hearing community, collectively comprise a community. And, most importantly, this community is bound together by its own language, American Sign Language (ASL). It is this duality of language systems (ASL of the deaf community and English of the hearing community) that provides the basis for this article.

As a result of this duality, the linguistic status of deaf people is a complex entity to describe. It may be helpful to begin by dividing the hearing-impaired community into three groups: (a) those deaf individuals who master ASL as a first language and English as a second language, (b) those who master English as a first language and ASL as a second language, and (c) those who master neither English nor ASL. The key word is *mastery*. Although, by loose definition, a large proportion of the deaf community can be characterized as bilingual (Haugen, 1977; Weinrich, 1953), the majority seldom achieve native mastery in either ASL or English. As a result, when an attempt is made to describe the linguistic status of a hearing-impaired young adult, the duality must be accounted for.

LANGUAGE DOMAIN OF DEAF YOUNG ADULTS

The concept of bilingual language users in the deaf community has been described by Stokoe (1970). Although the English element in the deaf person's language domain has long been recognized, it has only been recently that ASL has come to be recognized as a language (Klima & Bellugi, 1980; Stokoe, 1960; Stokoe, Casterline, & Croneberg, 1976).

Stokoe (1970) has suggested that there is a continuum of language usage in the ASL-English bilingual community between ASL and English. Woodward (1973) has further described a contact dialect between English and ASL. The dialect neither adheres strictly to English nor to ASL. Woodward calls the contact language *Pidgin Signed English* (PSE). Woodward and Reilly and McIntire (1978) discussed certain characteristics of PSE and compare them to their equivalent ASL and English constructions. It is this continuum of language usage to which a person attempting to assess the language domain of hearing-impaired persons must attend.

The difficulty with such a continuum representation lies in the fact that ASL and English are not polar opposites. Each language represents a continuum itself from a high level of skill to little or no skill. It should be pointed out that the ASL domain represents a range from competent ASL abilities to no knowledge of ASL. Thus, the range would include those who do not know ASL to those who sign ASL proficiently. The English range includes those who have a high level of proficiency in English to those who have little or no English skill. The domain of language for most deaf young adults is the result of an interaction between English competency and ASL competency. Given the complexity of this interactive model, can a reasonably accurate picture of the language abilities of the hearing-impaired young adults be established?

For practical purposes, there are, in fact, four possible configurations of ability depending on the particular language skills of the deaf person. The first type is the person who is proficient in both English and ASL and can fully interact in either language system, assuming that the channel used for their communication is open to both users. (A profoundly hearing-impaired person cannot be expected to use speech and listening as a channel, but reading, writing, and signing in English may be appropriate.) The second type is represented by the person who has a high level of skill in one language but no skill in the other. This person is monolingual and must be evaluated as such. The third type is a person who has a high level of skill in one language but moderate to low skill in the other language. The fourth type is the individual who knows some of each language but is not proficient in either. The task of assessing language abilities of hearing-impaired young adults is to establish a level of functioning within these domains.

ASSESSING LANGUAGE SKILLS

From earlier discussion, it might be unreasonable to assume that a deaf individual scoring at an eighth-grade level on a standardized test would behave linguistically like a hearing 13-year-old performing at grade level. It follows that a simple grade equivalency score on a language test would provide little information concerning how a particular deaf individual approaches a linguistic task. Furthermore, it has been suggested that standardized tests yield spuriously high scores for deaf students (Moores, 1971). It seems, then, what is necessary is a better diagnostic approach to evaluating a deaf individual's English performance beyond mere comprehension of grammatical and semantic structure on a standardized test. What is needed is a multifaceted assessment approach to evaluating the language competencies of individual hearing-impaired persons. Three broad areas must be included in any language assessment of hearing-impaired individuals: vocabulary, syntax, and experiential level.

Vocabulary

Assessment of vocabulary skills has always been linked to language skill development, especially in reading comprehension and general IQ development. Consider the inclusion of separate vocabulary tests in batteries such as the California Achievement Tests (Tiegs & Clark, 1963), Gates McGinitie Tests (Gates & McGinitie, 1965), and the Stanford Achievement Tests (Kelly et al., 1964), as well as their inclusion in individual intelligence tests such as the Stanford Binet and Wechsler scales. Use of such standardized measures with hearing-impaired individuals has continually demonstrated that the average hearing-impaired high school graduate scores at a level similar to that of a hearing 4th grader (Cooper & Rosenstein, 1966; DiFrancesca, 1972; Trybus & Karchmer, 1977).

Even though there is much norm-referenced data to support the handicapping effects of severe to profound hearing impairment on English vocabulary development, little research exists that details the nature of the vocabulary difficulty for the hearing-impaired students. To specifically define the nature or extent of vocabulary deficiency is not a simple task.

The first step in evaluating vocabulary must be to determine which words an individual knows. This is not an easy task. If one examines the traditional word frequency counts such as those by Thorndike and Lorge (1944), Kučera and Francis (1967), and Carroll, Davies, and Richman (1971), it becomes immediately evident that these lists contain a great deal of redundacy by using derivatives, inflections, compounds, and so on. Add to this the presence of function words, such as *the* (the most frequently occurring word in English), *a*, *but*, *that*, and *is*, and the size of the lexicon expands beyond just content words. Although knowledge of the words falling into the function class is important for achieving competence in language, the meaning of a word is difficult to assess outside of a syntactic context. Therefore, as a starting point a method of defining contentive words for measurement purposes is important to know.

From an English perspective, Durphy (1974) has provided a definition of a basic root word, which excludes proper nouns, derivatives, inflections, compounds, archaic words, foreign words, and technical terms. As a result, he has demonstrated that there must be about 12,000 basic words in English. He has extended his work to show that the average high school senior knows about 7,000 of these words, and the average student at the end of the third grade knows about 2,000 of these basic words. It would seem logical, especially for hearing-impaired students, that the development of an English vocabulary is related to the amount of visual exposure (through print and finger spelling) they have had with the lexicon. The same is true with sign language. The more exposure the student has had to the signs and their referents, the larger the usable vocabulary in that system will be. Regardless of the language system under consideration, a first step in evaluating a vocabulary must be to determine which words an individual knows.

However, complete evaluation of vocabulary skill does not end here. The ability of an individual to apply morphemic rules greatly expands the size of a working vocabulary. When one starts with the basic words in a person's vocabulary and adds the dimension of morphological knowledge, vocabulary ability is greatly improved. For this reason a complete assessment of vocabulary skill must entail an evaluation of a student's ability to employ morphological rules to his or her working basic vocabulary.

From an assessment point of view, it is probably not necessary to evaluate each of the morphological extensions that is possible for any given vocabulary word. However, two things are necessary: assessment of which of the basic root words is understood and assessment of knowledge of the morphological rules that can be applied to these words. Since there is considerable consistency in the way morphology is dealt with in language, this element can be assessed independently and inferences can be made concerning the ability of the student to apply the rules given knowledge of a basic root word. With such information in mind about a student, the

Another area of vocabulary assessment that must be considered is that of word flexibility.

---

teacher can make some judgments as to the abilities the student has in using various basic words in a language context.

Another area of vocabulary assessment that must be considered is that of word flexibility. For example, in English, given the same graphical form, *run*, can a student understand the meaning of *run* when printed in each of the following sentences?

- There has been a run on paper towels.
- She will run in the race.
- The president will run for re-election.
- A new house can run a lot of money.
- We have some errands to run this afternoon.
- Some dyes have a tendency to run.

Such flexibility in vocabulary usage is the key to comprehending printed messages. Again, using a basic word list such as that given previously (Durphy, 1974), it would be an important part of any vocabulary assessment to know how a student can use a given graphical form in a variety of contexts.

For the reasons described earlier, we do not advocate the use of norm-referenced tests to evaluate vocabulary skills. Such tests give little information about what students know and where they are having difficulty with the English lexicon. We suggest a three-dimensional approach to vocabulary assessment. The first accounts for basic, or root word, knowledge; the second, the morphological ability of the student; and the third, the ability to use words in a flexible manner in different parts of speech and with a variety of meanings. With such assessment knowledge an instructor or diagnostician can then determine what instruction must be provided and how long the road to remediation will be.

Syntax

The second area that must be assessed to gain information about language competency is the knowledge a person has about the syntax of the language system. The problem, however, is to develop a test to evaluate each of the individual structures that exist in any given language. Since the syntactic structure of a language is complex, it is not usually possible to test all structures given the constraints of space and time. The only realistic approach to assessing such skills is to sample a set of syntactic structures and develop a technique to evaluate these structures. Thus, the first step in attempting to measure syntactic abilities is to choose those syntactic categories that are appropriate for the instructional task at hand. As a result, the diagnostician must be judicious in making a choice, selecting those structures that will be representative. When using a test on syntactic abilities, the teacher must be aware of exactly what is being measured. If one is preparing questions about relativization, there must be an awareness of the different forms relativization can take. To evaluate only one or two forms might result in overgeneralization of the student's abilities, thus missing input in some needed area of instruction. For example, hearing-impaired students generally perform much better with relativization using *who* forms than with *that* forms.

It is impossible, within the limits of this article, to completely define the structure of any language system. It might even be questionable whether such a description has yet been completely documented. This is especially true for ASL. (For further reading in the area of English, the interested individual is referred to Akmajian & Heny, 1975; Bresnan, 1978; Stockwell, Schacter, & Partee, 1973. For ASL, to Klima & Bellugi, 1980; Stokoe et al., 1976; and Supalla & Newport, 1978, keeping in mind that these are various analyses of ASL, collectively comprising an incomplete grammar of ASL.)

By referring to the above sources, one should be able to determine the structures that will point the direction along which assessment in syntactic areas can proceed. Measurement of syntax without a clear-cut direction should not be attempted.

Experiential level

In addition to the traditionally emphasized vocabulary building and syntactic understanding as the important components of the curriculum, social context and the experience the individual brings to a language-learning situation also bear on the development of that individual's language skills (Ervin-Tripp, 1968). The role of experience is usually assumed, and its contribution to being a competent user of any language is seldom systematically considered during instruction. For most hearing students who already implicitly know the rules of the English language and have a relative large vocabulary, the nature of the content used in instruction is probably relatively minor. Such may not be true for the severe and profoundly hearing-impaired person.

Experience is best defined as that body of information that students bring with them to the learning activity. It is all of the stored information about the content used in the exercise and should incorporate such things as space–time relationships, reality versus fantasy, significance, interrelationships, and so on. In a sense, it is the way individuals order their world and the relationships among persons, places, and events.

If experience is so vital, then instructors in language should constantly be asking themselves, "Will the material I am using to evaluate language skills inhibit the language usage of my students?" Are you, as a teacher, expecting them to produce language about content for which they have no adequate basis of knowledge?

It must be remembered that much of the information that hearing learners take in comes through audition and reading. We depend heavily on these modes, but it is just these avenues of communication with which the hearing-impaired person has difficulty. One must always question whether it is *language* being measured or the student's *world knowledge*. We are so often concerned about syntactic and vocabulary levels that we seldom stop to consider whether the content is within the individual's level of comprehension. This question is fundamental to all areas of assessment, and must be given attention any time one sets out to evaluate skill levels in language.

EDUCATIONAL IMPLICATIONS OF INFORMATION ABOUT THE LANGUAGE DOMAIN

Although gathering information concerning the linguistic competency of individuals is important, there must be some end to which this information will assist the teacher or diagnostician in developing instructional plans. From the model presented earlier, it is clear that a good understanding of the particular language system(s) in which a student is operating is important. One must know the student's competencies in English as well as in ASL. To try to remediate one language without knowledge of the impact of the other can result in confusion on the part of both the language specialist and the student.

A key issue in any language instruction requires that the student be given a good model of the target language. Consider, for example, the teaching of English to the severe and profoundly hearing impaired when the individual may not be able to perceive auditorialy or visually the significant parts of the language's morphology or syntax. Although signing in exact English (incorporating all morphological units of English) may be one possible solution, it must be pointed out that only a person highly competent in sign language and English can hope to provide a model that will be perceived correctly by the hearing-impaired person. It is seldom the case that a student in a total communication or oral classroom has the opportunity to receive an exact representation of the English

The second area in which information about the individual's language domain can be applied is in providing support services for the hearing-impaired individual.

language (Marmor & Petitto, 1979). Using sign language does not automatically guarantee that English will be perceived correctly. Only when the instructor has the competencies to evaluate the level of language sophistication of the student, his/her own sophistication, and the type of representation occurring in the classroom can one hope to begin altering the educational environment to provide adequate models of language.

The second area in which information about the individual's language domain can be applied is in providing support services for a hearing-impaired individual. Even though it seems ludicrous, it may be that a student is being provided support services (e.g., tutoring, note-taking, or sign language services) and yet not have the prerequisite skills to be able to adequately use these services. Although it is good to provide support services directly to hearing-impaired individuals, it is quite another thing to ensure that these support services are maximizing the interactions that occur with the hearing-impaired individual. To provide a tutor who does not understand the English level of the individual or to provide a sign language interpreter whose sign language is far above the abilities of the individuals will have only minimal pay off in supporting the learning environment. Thus an understanding of the student's language domain can help in choosing staff and in providing the services to the hearing-impaired individual. An excellent reference for providers of support services can be found in Bishop (1979). This book presents practical ways for supporting the education of hearing-impaired students in the mainstreamed environment.

The nature of the ASL language system needs to be further defined so that appropriate instrumentation can be developed. Appropriate and realistic goals for remediation follow from a determination of the competency level of a student's language domain.

Another area that needs development is providing materials that draw on the language strengths of the deaf person. There are too few materials available for teaching English that take advantage of the student's understanding of ASL. Nor are there adequate materials for trying to teach English as a nonauditory system. Remember that English is a nonauditory language for most severe to profoundly hearing-impaired individuals.

REFERENCES

Akmajian, H., & Heny, F. *An introduction to the principles of transformational syntax.* Cambridge, Mass.: MIT Press, 1975.

Bishop, M.E. (Ed.). *Mainstreaming: Practical ideas for educating hearing-impaired students.* Washington, D.C.: A. G. Bell Association for the Deaf, 1979.

Bochner, J. Error, anomaly, and variation in the English of deaf individuals. *Language and Speech,* 1978, *21,* 174-189.

Bresnan, J. A realistic transformational grammar. In M. Halle, J. Bresnan, & G. Miller (Eds.), *Linguistic theory and psychological reality.* Cambridge, Mass.: MIT Press, 1978.

Carroll, J.B., Davies, P., & Richman, B. *Word frequency book.* Boston: Houghton Mifflin, 1971.

Cooper, R.L., & Rosenstein, J. Language acquisition of deaf children. *Volta Review,* 1966, *68,* 58–67.

DiFrancesca, S. *Academic achievement test results of a national testing program for hearing impaired students: United States, spring, 1971.* Washington, D.C.: Gallaudet College, Office of Demographic Studies, 1972.

Durphy, H.F. *The rationale, development and standardization of a basic word vocabulary test.* (DHEW Publication No. HRA 74-1334). Washington, D.C.: U.S. Government Printing Office, 1974.

Ervin-Tripp, S. An analysis of the interaction of language, topic and listener. In J. Fishman (Ed.), *Readings in sociology of language.* The Hague, The Netherlands: Mouton, 1968.

Gates, H.I., & McGinitie, W.I. *Gates McGinitie Reading Tests.* New York: Teachers College Press, 1965.

Haugen, E., Norm and deviation in bilingual communities. In P. Hornby (Ed.), *Bilingualism: Psychological, social, and educational implications.* New York: Academic Press, 1977.

Kelly, T., Madden, R., Gardner, E., & Rudman, H. *Stanford Achievement Tests—Advanced Battery.* New York: Harcourt, Brace & World, 1964.

Klima, E., & Bellugi, U. *The signs of language.* Cambridge, Mass.: Harvard University Press, 1980.

Kučera, H., & Francis, W. *Computational analysis of present day American English.* Providence, R.I.: Brown University Press, 1967.

Marmor, G.S., & Petitto, L. Simultaneous communication in the classroom: How well is English grammar represented? *Sign Language Studies,* 1979, *23,* 99–136.

Moores, D.F. Psycholinguistics and deafness. *American Annals of the Deaf,* 1970, *115,* 37–48.

Moores, D.F. *An investigation of the psycholinguistic functioning of deaf adolescents* (Research Rep. No. 18). Minneapolis: University of Minnesota, Research and Development Center in Education of Handicapped Children, 1971.

Reilly, J. & McIntire, M.L. ASL and PSE: What's the difference? Unpublished manuscript, California State University, Northridge, 1978.

Sarachan-Deily, A.B., & Love, R.J. Underlying grammatical rule structure in the deaf. *Journal of Speech and Hearing Research,* 1974, *17,* 689–698.

Schlesinger, H.S., & Meadow, K.P. *Deafness and mental health: A developmental approach.* San Francisco: Langley Porter Institute, 1971.

Stockwell, R.R., Schacter, P., & Partee, B.H. *The major*

syntactic structures of English. New York: Holt, Rinehart, & Winston, 1973.

Stokoe, W. Sign language structure: An outline of the visual communication systems of the American deaf. *Studies in linguistics.* University of Buffalo, Occasional Paper No. 8, 1960.

Stokoe, W.C. Sign language diglossia. *Studies in Linguistics,* 1970, *21,* 27–41.

Stokoe, W., Casterline, D. & Croneberg, G. *A dictionary of American Sign Language on linguistic principles.* Washington, D.C.: Gallaudet College Press, 1976.

Supalla, T. & Newport. E. How many seats in a chair? The derivation of nouns and verbs in American Sign Language. In P. Siple (Ed.), *Understanding language through sign language research.* New York: Academic Press, 1978.

Swisher, L. The language performance of the oral deaf. In H. Whitaker & H. A. Whitaker (Eds.), *Studies in neurolinguistics* (Vol. 2). New York: Academic Press, 1976.

Tiegs, E.W., & Clark, W.W. *California Reading Tests.* Monterey, Calif.: California Test Bureau, 1963.

Trybus, R.J., & Karchmer, M.A. School achievement scores of hearing-impaired children: National data on achievement status and growth patterns. *American Annals of the Deaf,* 1977, *122,* 62–69.

Tweeny, K.S., & Hoemann, H.W. The development of semantic associations in profoundly deaf children. *Journal of Speech and Hearing Research,* 1973, *16,* 309–318.

Thorndike, L.L. & Lorge, I. *The teachers word book of 30,000 words.* New York: Bureau of Publications, Teachers College, Columbia University, 1944.

Weinrich, U. *Languages in contact.* New York: Linguistic Circle of New York, 1953.

Woodward, J. Some characteristics of Pidgin Sign English. *Sign Language Studies,* 1973, *3,* 39–46.

Societal forces influencing the roles of speech-language pathologists, audiologists, and teachers of the deaf

E. Harris Nober, PhD
Department of Communication Disorders
University of Massachusetts
Amherst, Massachusetts

AS WE REVIEW the literature in the field of language disorders, we inevitably learn of the advocacy role of parents of hearing-impaired children. Historically and currently, groups of professionals and parents have lobbied for legislation to alter services so that handicapped individuals can enjoy equal educational opportunity. Groups representing hearing-impaired children have been and continue to be in the forefront of such efforts.

Major controversies and concerns remain among parents and professionals. The issues present difficulties for program planners, service providers, and training programs. As increasing numbers of hearing-impaired students are served in regular education settings, formidable questions about appropriate services emerge. As an attempt is made to determine the effective balance of services, we rely on a historic and thematic overview of the growth of the fields of language intervention for the hearing impaired. The threads

0271-8294/82/0023-0076$2.00
© 1982 Aspen Systems Corporation

of speech–language pathology, audiology, education of the deaf, linguistics, child development, reading, and psychology as fields of study and professions are herein reviewed revealing both biases and philosophical underpinnings.

A HISTORICAL PERSPECTIVE

Complimenting the educational and remedial developments revolving around deafness during the past several decades has been the basic research at the universities in general semantics, experimental phonetics, language development, and linguistics. Clearly, scientific methodology and research techniques were being facilitated by this "scientific" community. In some instances, private industry (i.e., RCA, Bell Telephone) contributed significantly to communication research).

Early advances

An interesting marker for the profession occurred in 1914 when Smiley Blanton, a Cornell University speech instructor, completed a medical degree. Blanton was hired by the University of Wisconsin to set up the first speech clinic in the United States. In 1921 Wisconsin awarded Sara Stinchfield the first PhD and Robert West the second. West remained at Wisconsin and audited medical classes to propagate the strong medical orientation of Wisconsin. At the University of Iowa, there was a stronghold in psychology and general semantics under the chair of Carl Seashore. In 1923 Iowa set up a speech correction clinic and hired Lee Travis and Jack Wendell Johnson. Other universities also started programs by hiring young scientists: Columbia University had Scripture; the University of Pennsylvania, Troutmeyer; the University of Illinois, Giles Gray; Ohio State University, G. Oscar Russell; the University of Michigan, Edwin Myskens; and Princeton University, Ernest Glen Wever.

Dissemination outlets for the research were limited, but one outlet was the National Association of Teachers of Speech, an association that had grown large and then factionated into enclaves. One group consisting of speech correctionists agitated for its own publication, and on December 29, 1925, a group of 11 speech-correction scholars headed by West founded the American Academy of Speech Correction.

The history and growth of professional organizations evolved as an interdependent matrix governed by the economic, political, and social forces of the times. The turbulent years of the 1920s gave rise to the turbulent but determined beginnings of these associations. It took high goals and hard work to establish a momentum to survive the 1930s with the Depression and 18% unemployment. Unemployment for professionals would have been worse if President Roosevelt had not intervened with special employment for scholars. Halfway through this decade, Congress passed the 1935 Social Security Act, which was amended to include disability insurance for disabled workers, using up to 1.5% of its trust fund. This represented the hallmark of public assistance programs for the disabled and handicapped relative to vocational employment.

During the 1930s texts on communication disorders appeared; terminology was established based on psychology, medicine, general semantics, experimental psychology, engineering, education, research methodology, and so on; considerable normative data were collated; and instrumentation was constantly appearing. Research papers mostly dealt with stuttering, and the rest were about articulation, organic speech disorders, voice, and so forth. Dorothy McCarthy (1930) described the language development of preschool children, an extension of Piaget's (1926) treatise on the language and thought of the child. Irene Poole (1934) produced her often-quoted study on the genetic development of articulation and consonant sounds.

> *Inflated expectations that hearing loss and psychogenic hearing impairment would result from war trauma led to the establishment of several aural rehabilitation and diagnostic centers throughout the country.*

Orton (1937), a physician, related cerebral dominance to language disorders. Not until the end of the decade did Max Goldstein (1939) publish his famous acoustic method of training the deaf and hard of hearing.

The 1940s were consumed by World War II and its wake. Interest in language expanded and diversified abruptly. Stuttering research and clinical service continued to predominate, but articulation therapy research accelerated and the research on language disorders concentrated on adult aphasia because of the war. The interface between psychologists and neurologists generated the writings of Wepman, Eisenson, Halstead, and Goldstein.

Inflated expectations that hearing loss and psychogenic hearing impairment (pseudohypacusis) would result from war trauma led to the establishment of several aural rehabilitation and diagnostic centers throughout the country (e.g., Deshon, Borden, Hoff, Philadelphia Naval Station, Veterans Administration hospitals) and an outstanding federally funded research team assembled at the Harvard Psychoacoustic Laboratory (PAL). In part, the PAL research provided the underpinning for the emerging field of audiology.

The evolution of audiology also hinged on the framework provided by the otologic community and physiologists like Wever, Bray, Bekesy, and Bell Telephone scientists. Indeed, the medical component still claims Norton Canfield as the father of audiology, whereas others claim Raymond Carhart.

Considerable progress also occurred in regard to the handicapped in general. In 1943, Grace Fernald founded her famous remedial clinic for children in California. The classic maturational and developmental indices of infants and children of Arnold Gesell (a physician) were published in the middle of the decade. But the hallmark work was the Alfred Strauss and Laura Lehtinen (1947) classic *Psychopathology and Education of the Brain-Injured Child*. Borderline children previously labeled as mentally retarded, emotionally disturbed, autistic, aphasic, behaviorly maladjusted, hyperkinetic, and so on, were touted as minimally brain injured. Strauss and Lehtinen pioneered and developed the use of psychomotor tests, classifying behavioral symptoms, perceptual manifestations, and psychometric indices.

During this decade there was considerable progress in programs for the hearing impaired. A number of tests for speech reading were developed. Research on the psychological aspect of deafness in children evolved. In England, Ewing and Ewing (1947) published on deaf education, amplification, and early assessment.

The 1950s

During the 1950s, Congress passed the Cooperative Research Act to foster gainful research between the federal government and universities. Two thirds of the funds were earmarked for mental retardation. In 1958, the launching of Sputnik led to a bonanza of federal aid to education for research and development centers, government-supported programs, money for the handicapped (the Kennedy interest in mental retardation), jobs for professionally trained people, and support funds for student trainees. Spinoffs from the space research programs led to the transistor, electronic miniaturization to be used in audiometry, hearing aids, computers, and research equipment. Training programs erupted throughout the country, with expensive sound suites and equipment being charged to federal agencies along with the personnel and student trainees to complete the package.

On the sociological scene the authoritarian orientation indigenous to the 1940s (war protocol and Freudian theory) succumbed to the permissive individualization of the 1950s. There was wide acceptance of the "self," and in therapy stutterers were encouraged to accept their difference and to stutter more efficiently. Self-testing and self-directed decision making led to an eruption of encounter groups, with people sharing problems and a reward system more concerned with the willful attempt toward remediation rather than a successful performance. The movement to individualization transformed remedial therapy conducted in groups to a one-on-one format. In education, success became relative to the individual and much less absolute, hence the criterion-referenced model of assessment emerged. Clearly, norms became less intimidating. Objectivity became a catchword, a way of plucking things out of context. Objectivity had multiple meanings, and in audiology there was the race for objective hearing tests, among other things. Thus, an individual could remain passive while electroencephalogram electrodes scanned the central nervous system or the galvanic skin response electrodes tuned into the autonomic nervous system.

During the 1950s otosurgery and cleft palate reconstructive surgery were advanced, with remedial success often dependent on surgical intervention. Otosurgery achieved miraculous proportions.

During this decade, inroads evolved for the understanding of speech and language development and disorders in children (McCarthy, 1959; Mowrer, 1952). There were Licklider and Miller's (1953) "Perception of Speech," Stevens and Davis's (1954) *Hearing: Its Psychology and Physiology*, and numerous studies dealing with the psychology of deafness. Auditory training research made laudatory progress due to the work of Hudgins (1954) at the

Clarke School for the Deaf, Silverman at the Central Institute for the Deaf, Carhart at Northwestern University, and foreigners such as Wedenberg (1950), who reported on auditory training for severely hard-of-hearing school children. Frey and Whetnal (1954) published their auditory approach to training deaf children, and Ewing and Ewing (1947) continued their investigations on deafness. In 1954, Myklebust published his still-popular *Auditory Disorders in Children* and was preparing his *Psychology of Deafness* (1964) and learning disabilities monograph series for the next decade. At the molecular level, physiologists were relating neuron loss to auditory discrimination (Neff, 1958), and additional neurophysiological progress occurred with mental retardation, cerebral palsy, and aphasia.

The undisputed landmark feature of this decade was the classic work of Noam Chomsky (1957). Terminology changed drastically as the language process divided into phonology, syntax, and semantics. Most of all, the imposing biolinguistic frame of reference (Lenneberg, 1967) concerning language acquisition dwarfed all previous theories of language development.

The turbulent 1960s

From a professional perspective, the 1960s were turbulent. Social authoritarianism continued to erode as advocate groups assumed more responsibility at all societal levels. Accountability demands led to the further demise of authoritarianism. Parents and administrators required justification of programs with viable evidence of improvement and progress. Consumer protection and consumer rights were stressed. As a consequence a forceful, self-indulgent pride of the handicapped surfaced. Universities and governmental agencies set up human subjects committees to protect people against research exploitation; physicians were swamped with malpractice suits.

With regard to the handicapped, categorical labels were also modified as the movement toward cross categorization became popular. At one end of the continuum, all handicapped and disadvantaged children were designated as *special needs children*, and at the other end were the medical terms such as cerebral palsy and aphasic. Between the two ends were terms like *visually impaired, auditorally impaired, developmentally disabled, physically handicapped*, and *health impaired*, with intragrouping in some instances, such as mild–moderate–severe, high–incidence, low–incidence, and so on. Not infrequently, anyone left over with a learning or an attention deficit, hyperkinesis, impulsivity, minimal brain damage, perceptual deficits, or psychomotor differences was designated as *learning disabled*. Disadvantaged children were inadvertently included in the learning disabilities group until nondiscriminatory assessment was enforced as part of Public Law (PL) 94-142.

Educational and remedial management procedures went full orbit from drill to training to therapy to conditioning to behavior modification, with ongoing diagnoses refurbished as prescriptive teaching. Terms like *decision making* and *cost-effective* provided an aura of leadership capability for everyone to dabble with.

Marked progress occurred in all fields

that deal with handicapped children. McGinnis continued Fernald's work in language disorders and aphasia. Dunn, Cruickshank, Kirk, Frostig, Myklebust, Getman, Kephart, and others revamped the field of special education to what exists today, providing the hardware and software research support data that served as the bases for educational models. During the 1960s the learning problems of disadvantaged children were also addressed as cultural differences to be reckoned with.

Research on deafness took many directions: The student curriculum was improved, psychosocial effects of deafness were systematically studied, home programs were developed for parents, and amplification systems were revolutionized. The traditional gap separating teachers of the deaf and audiologists narrowed with the meeting of a joint committee on audiology, education of the deaf, and Bureau for the Education of Handicapped. Although federal training and research support increased during the 1950s, federal participation mushroomed in the 1960s and reached its zenith during the 1970s. Federal support financed the development of new training programs through the program assistance grants, research and innovation grants, state incentive grants, a media center on deafness, and so on. Older children and adults received federal support from other health-related groups (e.g., the National Institutes of Health; Social Rehabilitative Services; Administration, VA training programs, National Institute of Education, and the National Science Foundation).

Audiology underwent a major growth spurt during the 1960s. In 1966 the Academy of Rehabilitative Audiology was formed to establish a strong service-delivery component. Technology impacted to miniaturize the hearing aid as transistors and subsequently painted circuitry were perfected. As costs reduced, schools could indulge in more elaborate equipment. Computer technology, applied to neurophysiological measures, enabled audiometric tests to record cortical activity, subcortical brain stem activity, and eventually eighth nerve peripheral activity to auditory stimuli. Most of the basic research on impedance audiometry occurred during this decade. Surgical restoration of the middle ear was revolutionary.

Remedial therapy programs improved, with clear roles outlined for schools for the deaf, speech and hearing centers, local educational agencies (LEAs), and public school clinicians. Certification and accreditation agencies established coherent standards. Eventually, state educational agencies (SEAs) adopted licensure and teaching standards based on the requirements of the professional organizations, such as the American Speech–Language and Hearing Association (ASHA), Council for Exceptional Children (CEC), Conference of Executives of American Schools for the Deaf, (CEASD) and the Council on Education of the Deaf (CED).

LEGISLATION AND ENTITLEMENT PROGRAMS

A building momentum

The decade of the 1970s was perhaps the zenith for the handicapped. The black civil rights movement of the 1950s was followed in the 1960s by women's rights and in the 1970s with the rights of the handicapped.

PL 94-142 did not erupt out of a vacuum; indeed, it was nearly the 200th federal law dealing with handicapped persons or social entitlements. The history of governmental legislation for the handicapped began in 1823 when the first state school for the deaf was established in Kentucky. Ohio and other states quickly followed, but it was another 25 years before the U.S. Congress enacted additional legislation for the handicapped. Within 20 to 30 years, schools for the blind, mentally retarded, and other handicapped persons sprung up in New York, Boston, Philadelphia, Providence, and Hartford. In 1857 Congress established the first federal educational agency, the Columbia Institution for the Instruction of the Deaf and Dumb and the Blind (PL 35-39), which was renamed Gallaudet College in 1954 (PL 83-420). By the end of the 1800s, there were about 14 federal laws to aid the handicapped, each having improved and expanded entitlements.

Since rehabilitation of the disabled was not construed to be a federal responsibility, it was not until 1918 that the World War I Soldier's Vocational Rehabilitation Act (PL 65-178) was enacted to provide disabled veterans with vocational rehabilitation. This was followed by the Citizens Vocational Rehabilitation Act in 1920 to service nonveterans (PL 66-236). In 1943, the Citizens Act added the mentally retarded and emotionally disturbed (PL 78-113). Amendments were added in 1954 (PL 83-565); in 1961 (PL 87-276) for research, demonstration, and training; and in 1967 for a National Commission on Architectural Barriers and the National Center for Deaf–Blind Youth (PL 89-105). Soon afterward came Medicaid and Medicare programs for the disabled. Between 1920 and 1959 another 51 laws adding benefits and entitlements were passed. Although handicapped legislation was scattered, it was President Kennedy who facilitated a national plan for studying mental retardation and other anomalies.

A milestone enactment in 1965 was PL 89-10, the Elementary and Secondary Education Act (ESEA), which supplemented LEA programs for educationally deprived children. Then came PL 89-313 and its Title I program. A plethora of federal legislative acts occurred during the 1960s, including creation of the National Technical Institute for the Deaf; Mental Retardation and Mental Health and Community Health Center construction acts; extended federal assistance acts for state-operated and state-supported schools for the handicapped; the Vocational Rehabilitation Act (PL 89-333) and its amendments; the Model Secondary School for Deaf Act (PL 89-694), with amendments to the Elementary and Secondary Education Act; the National Eye Institute; the Handicapped Children Early Education Assistance Act (PL 90-538); the National Center in Educational Media for Handicapped (PL 91-61). During this decade, 54 laws relative to the handicapped were enacted.

The zenith: the 1970s

The decade of the 1970s may turn out to be the peak of the century. During the first 5 years, 61 enactments were passed, making a total of 115 for the 15-year span. In 1973 came PL 93-112, the Vocational Rehabilitation Act. It prioritized services, added joint client-counselor decision-making policy, and prohibited discrimination. Congress amended the ESEA (PL 93-380) by increasing funds from $100 million to $660 million plus guarantees for due process, least restrictive environment, and state goal commitments, including timetables for full educational opportunities for all handicapped and gifted children.

The culminating legislation was the Education for All Handicapped Children Act (PL 94-142), a revision of Part B of the prior Education of the Handicapped Act (PL 91-230). PL 94-142, often called the human rights bill for handicapped children, has affected and altered all levels of student training preparation and direct service delivery. It mandated accountability, family involvement, due process, free and appropriate education, and nondiscriminatory assessment; included all handicapped children ages 3–21 years; provided for individual educational planning using teams comprising parents or advocates, funding schedules, and a schedule of responsibilities for SEAs and LEAs; required vendors to be well-trained and competent; was self-contained; required in-service programs; espoused a least-restrictive-environment educational model; and defined handicapped prototypes. The bill impacted heavily on all phases of educational management of handicapped children, and no institution, group, or agency was spared. In an effort to comply, a massive cooperative effort occurred among agencies; consortiums and collaboratives became commonplace throughout the country.

During the 1970s technological advances nearly automated some phases of diagnostic audiometry. Impedance audiometry became so universal that it is now a standard school tool. Hearing aid fidelity and other amplification systems continued to improve. The coveted aural/oral model in educational management for the deaf was giving ground to the total approach. Even more brazen in scope was the commitment to the alternative language orientation for the nonverbal. Some of the alternative language techniques were enhanced by the revolutionization of computer technology by microprocessor chips in the 1980s. During the 1970s neurophysiological inroads were marked. During this decade research on the hearing impaired concentrated on alternative educational models, psychology of deafness, language development issues, sign language, public access of the handicapped to public institutions, state licensure codes, certification and accreditation, in-service and continuing educational opportunities for persons serving the handicapped, and new diagnostic and assessment instruments.

The reluctantly relinquished privileges

Federal legislation inflated government entitlements to such an extent that nearly everyone, rich or poor, normal or handicapped, adult or child, was potentially some sort of entitlement beneficiary.

given to special interest groups, minorities, the handicapped, and the elderly in the 1950s and 1960s became the rights of these groups by the 1970s. Federal legislation inflated government entitlements to such an extent that nearly everyone, rich or poor, normal or handicapped, adult or child, was potentially some sort of entitlement beneficiary. During the 1970s the cost of living rose 138% and entitlement programs more than quadrupled from $70 billion to $295 billion in the United States.

The future

It is conceivable that the intellectual surge of the 1970s may not totally survive the tempered 1980s. Plans have already been formulated to reduce space programs and their technological spinoffs, to reduce supplemented federal assistance to schools, college tuition loans, social security, health benefits, and so on. Even the recently established U.S. Department of Education with cabinet level status is to be downgraded to office or institute status.

It is fair to prognosticate what the effects of federal cutbacks in programs will be. Research will continue at a less accelerated pace but will be supplemented with more private industry and university interface. Microprocessor technology will progress geometrically and soon impact on daily living and educational management. Indeed, computer programs are already available for the handicapped with assist speech and language modules. Since most innovative classrooms will have microprocessor computer units, remedial education for the handicapped may become more self-directed and based on a competency strategy.

Technology will impact on surgical and medical management to produce a longer life span, which will precipitate more geriatric problems and an improvement in prosthetic devices. Educational programs will be predicated with increased SEA control due to federal block funding. Indeed, even PL 94-142 is being revised in a congressional subcommittee. During the decade, longitudinal data regarding PL 94-142 are sure to emerge concerning the effects and efficiency of mainstreaming or toward the least restrictive environment. The teacher training curriculum will include modules on serving the handicapped, so specialists will have smaller direct service roles in the total education of the handicapped and the underprivileged. Also, progress in the neurological areas, due to computerized tomography scan and similar innovations, should result in improved understanding of the neurologically impaired child.

TRAINING BASE

Prior to the 1800s, physicians, teaching monks, and philosophers explored their own informal techniques and demonstrated them. Early organizations mostly consisted of the handicapped and their parents. Paradoxically, the deaf groups were the most vocal; they organized for social, economic, and political benefits and were forceful in generating legislative mandates. Eventually, professional groups espoused the same causes and formed advocate groups in the crusade for better conditions. Curiously, the term *learning disabilities* resulted during a discussion in a joint meeting of a parent group and several invited professionals.

Professional organizations expanded their vistas as they grew in size, and many became involved with accreditation, certification, and licensure procedures and standards at federal, state, institutional, and individual levels. Standards established by a given group seemed to endure a 20-year longevity before the cumulative changes of the period precipitated revision and strengthening. Requirements became more specialized with each standards modification to foster more expertise and competence.

Even though nearly 50% to 70% of the graduates of speech and language pathology and audiology programs will gravitate to the school sector, academic personnel preparation requirements often do not require courses in special education or classroom teaching. Blanchard and Nober (1978) researched the impact of state and federal legislation on school speech–language and hearing clinicians before and after legislation. Skills were grouped under identification, evaluation, administration, and education. Clinicians indicated that after PL 94-142 was enacted, several skills assumed greater importance, for example, screening, preparing behavioral objectives, outlining individual educational plans, serving as case manager, team decision making, and preschool intervention strategies. Some of the notable case load additions were the hearing impaired, multiply handicapped, language disordered, developmentally delayed, and children with neurogenic pathologies. Clinicians depicted themselves as more visible in the total service delivery process and more directly accountable to administrators, parents, and professionals. Job roles, now more closely integrated into the general educational arena, included in-service responsibilities, core team evaluations, and community services. Curiously, direct service contacts dropped 25%, but an equal percentage of clinicians were hired to meet service needs.

The Council on Education of the Deaf (CED) standards present an interesting contrast to those of ASHA. ASHA standards emphasize the clinician, whereas CED standards are geared to teacher or instructional personnel preparation; the latter are expected to have a broad general knowledge of the field and expertise in one area of specialization. The bachelor's degree is a minimal requirement for the CED; the master's (or equivalent) is minimal for ASHA. The CED competencies include skills to identify and evaluate educational problems from infancy through adulthood. Specialization areas include preprimary, elementary, secondary, academic or special subjects, multiply handicapped, and special content areas.

A counterpart of the CED specialist could be the educational audiologist, but there are extremely few, if any, states that have allocated specific educational audiology clinical or teaching lines. Educational audiologists are employed in schools for the deaf, and some public school programs have hired them as speech–language clinicians who provide audiological services to hearing-impaired children. Clearly, there is no identifiable professional area that runs parallel to the speech clinician or the teacher of hearing-impaired children.

Professionals have noted that even a mild hearing loss in school children can delay receptive and expressive communication. Hence, there will be an impact on self-concept and social interaction and not infrequently a diminution of learning efficiency when a language deficit is involved. It is becoming apparent that if the educational audiologist is to coexist with the other specialists, skills will have to include competencies for overall comprehensive educational management of hearing-impaired children. A recent (August 1981) statement prepared by an ad hoc committee of ASHA addressing comprehensive audiology services in the schools listed prevention, identification, assessment, rehabilitation and instructional services, follow-up, referral and monitoring, technical assistance, administrative support, evaluation, and research. The report contended that the needs of hearing-impaired children are so diverse that only a team effort can hope to serve the child effectively and further asserted that including an audiologist on the team would "discourage overemphasis on the medical aspects of hearing impairment" and facilitate appropriate intervention. Also outlined were four general models to direct audiologic services into the school system:

- a parent-referral model
- a school-based/self-contained model
- a school- and community-based model
- a contractual agreement model.

It is safe to conjecture that in the current decade, the training base and competencies of audiologists and teachers of the hearing-impaired will be brought into closer focus. Considerably more overlap in scope may be required to adequately serve the hearing impaired in the school setting.

WHAT LIES AHEAD?

As indicated earlier, the history of professional and social activities relative to handicapped children interact with current events at all societal levels. Predicting the trends of the future for educating handicapped children is tantamount to predicting the parameters of the future, that is, world events, national politics; technological innovations; medical, genetic, and biophysiological advancements, and so on. One thing is certain: Progress is imminent; ongoing changes are often imperceptible, often jolting, the cumulative product is enduring. Overall progress rarely regresses; semantics alone precludes this. Hence, technology will continue to advance, medicine will move forward in cadence with technology and biochemistry, people will insist on a forceful determination of their own destiny, and the handicapped will demand quality treatment and dedicated commitment.

The only personnel preparation training program for the handicapped that will be noteworthy as a model program is one that propels the pack forward. Its graduates will need to understand and manipulate exceptionality, be able to utilize incessantly changing technology, and work in unison with other related professional workers. Clearly, ASHA requirements should include more areas that stress teaching skill and curriculum design, now emphasized in the CED standards. Conversely, CED requirements should recognize the medical and research focus of ASHA. It is entirely possible that some areas of specialty will fuse, leaving significantly blurred specialty delineations. The future teacher of the hearing-impaired child could be a doctoral-level specialist with the theoretical knowledge of a linguist, the clinical acumen of the speech–language pathologist–audiologist, the patience and optimism of a special educator with resource-room teacher endowments, and the program disipline of the remedial reading teacher with a powerful backlog of competencies.

Frankly, I look forward to the future and started to prepare for it when I entered the field three decades ago. It is the only way to stay on target and endure as an effective teacher of handicapped children. As long as I can recall, progress has always moved at an accelerated pace. I even recollect a time when reading only one professional journal kept the reader abreast of the field. No more—and this is perhaps the real testimony for future optimism.

REFERENCES

Blanchard, M., & Nober, E. H. The impact of state and federal legislation on public school speech language and hearing clinicians. *Language, Speech and Hearing Services in Schools*, 1978, 9(2), 77–84.

Chomsky, N. *Syntactic structures*. The Hague, The Netherlands: Mouton, 1957.

Ewing, I. E., & Ewing, A. G. *Opportunity and the deaf child*. London: University of London Press, 1947.

Fernald, G. *Remedial techniques in basic school subjects*. New York: McGraw-Hill, 1943.

Frey, D. B., & Whetnal, E. The auditory approach in training deaf children. *Lancet*, 1954, 266, 584–587.

Goldstein, M. *The acoustic method for the training of the deaf and hard-of-hearing child*. St. Louis, Mo.: Laryngoscope Press, 1939.

Hudgins, C. V. Auditory training: Its possibilities and limitations. *Volta Review*, 1954, 56, 1.

Lenneberg, E. *Biological foundations of language*. New York: Wiley, 1967.

Licklider, J. D. R., & Miller, G. Perception of speech. In S. S. Stevens (Ed.), *Handbook of experimental psychology*. New York: Wiley, 1953.

McCarthy, D. A. *Language development of the preschool child* (Institution of Child Welfare Monograph Series No. 4,). Minneapolis: University of Minnesota Press, 1930.

McCarthy, D. Research in language development: Retrospect and prospect. *Monograph of the Society for Research in Child Development*, 1959, 24, 3–24.

Mowrer, H. O. Speech development in the young child. *Journal of Speech and Hearing Disorders*, 1952, 17, 263–268.

Myklebust, H. R. *Auditory disorders in children: A manual for differential diagnosis*. New York: Grune & Stratton, 1954.

Myklebust, H. R. *The psychology of deafness* (2nd ed.). New York: Grune & Stratton, 1964.

Neff, W. D., Diamond, I. T. The neural basis of auditory discrimination. In H. F. Harlow & C. Woolsey (Eds.), *Biological and behavioral bases of behavior*. Madison: University of Wisconsin Press, 1958.

Orton, S. T. *Reading, writing and speech problems in children*. New York: Norton, 1937.

Piaget, J. *The language and thought of the child*. New York: Harcourt, Brace & World, 1926.

Poole, I. The genetic development of the articulation of consonant sounds. *Elementary English Review*, 1934, 9, 159–161.

Stevens, S. S., & Davis, H. *Hearing: Its psychology and physiology*. New York: Wiley, 1954.

Strauss, A., & Lehtinen L. *Psychopathology and education of the brain-injured child*. New York: Grune & Stratton, 1947.

Wedenberg, E. Auditory training of severely hard of hearing school children. *Acta Otolaryngologica*, 1950, Supplement 110, 1–82.

Notices

Notices featured in TLD include information on upcoming events and other areas of interest. Please address all material to be considered for publication in Notices to: Editor, Notices, TLD, Aspen Systems Corporation, 1600 Research Boulevard, Rockville, MD 20850.

INTERPRETERS FOR DEAF CONVENE IN HARTFORD

The National Registry of Interpreters for the Deaf (RID) will hold its biennial convention in Hartford, Connecticut, July 27 through August 1, 1982, at the Sheraton-Hartford Hotel. Details on the program are available from RID Convention 1982 Chairman, Christine Stranges, c/o Connecticut Registry of Interpreters for the Deaf, P.O. Box 12202, Hartford, Conn. 06112.

INTERNATIONAL CONFERENCE ON LEARNING DISABILITIES

October 7–9, 1982 is the date for the International Conference on Learning Disabilities, sponsored by the Council for Learning Disabilities to be held in Kansas City, Missouri. For further information contact: Gaye McNutt, CLD Executive Secretary, College of Education, University of Oklahoma, Norman, OK 73019.

GRADUATE ASSISTANTSHIPS

The University of Nevada, Las Vegas, is seeking qualified applicants for their master's degree program in Early Childhood Education for the Handicapped to apply for graduate assistantships. Assistantships include $5,000 for a 10-month contract for the academic year 1982–1983 and tuition waiver according to university regulations.

Requirements for graduate assistants include 20 hours of work per week related to the student's degree program. Qualifications include a bachelor's degree in an appropriate area with certification in special education, elementary education, or early childhood education.

For admissions and assistantship materials contact: James F. Adams, Dean, The Graduate College, University of Nevada, Las Vegas, Nevada 89154, (702) 736-3320. For further information about the program contact Nasim Dil, Director, Early Childhood Education for the Handicapped Training Program, College of Education, Room 112, University of Nevada, Las Vegas, Nevada 89154, (702) 736-3875.